D1331492

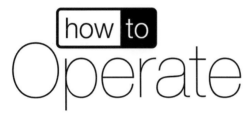

how to Operate

Matthew Stephenson
Surgical Registrar
South East Thames Rotation

WILEY-BLACKWELL

A John Wiley & Sons, Ltd., Publication

This edition first published 2011, © 2011 by John Wiley & Sons, Ltd

Wiley-Blackwell is an imprint of John Wiley & Sons, formed by the merger of Wiley's global Scientific, Technical and Medical business with Blackwell Publishing.

Registered office: John Wiley & Sons, Ltd, The Atrium, Southern Gate, Chichester, West Sussex, PO19 8SQ, UK

Editorial offices: 9600 Garsington Road, Oxford, OX4 2DQ, UK
The Atrium, Southern Gate, Chichester, West Sussex, PO19 8SQ, UK
111 River Street, Hoboken, NJ 07030-5774, USA

For details of our global editorial offices, for customer services and for information about how to apply for permission to reuse the copyright material in this book please see our website at www.wiley.com/wiley-blackwell.

The right of the author to be identified as the author of this work has been asserted in accordance with the UK Copyright, Designs and Patents Act 1988.

Library of Congress Cataloging-in-Publication Data is available for this title.
ISBN   978-0-470-65744-7

A catalogue record for this book is available from the British Library.

Set in 8.5/12pt HelveticaNeue by MPS Limited, a Macmillan Company, Chennai, India
Printed and bound in Singapore by Markono Print Media Pte Ltd

2   2012

Acknowledgments

Professional

There are so many people to thank and I apologise that I can't name everyone individually here. The biggest thanks have to go to the patients who without exception, were happy to be involved in this project to help develop surgical training.

- East Sussex NHS Trust, Brighton and Sussex University Hospitals NHS Trust, Medway NHS Foundation Trust and Eastbourne Downs Primary Care Trust at The Avenue for allowing the filming to take place at their marvellous institutions
- The operating consultants have all already been listed individually in the List of Contributors and I'm hugely grateful to each of them for participating so readily
- Sister Cheryl Funnell of the Conquest Hospital for illuminating us on many of the hidden secrets of theatre
- All of the scrub nurses and other theatre staff who were universally helpful in the process
- Sister Judith Wardale at Bexhill, Nicky Ward at Eastbourne and Siobhan O'Neill at the RSCH
- All the secretaries of the consultants for putting up with endless emails and phone calls, especially Stella Huggett, Helen Putman and Nina Lapier
- The waiting list officers at all sites, also for putting up with my unending phone calls
- Junior doctors James Jack, Phakanant Chaichanavichkij and Catherine Stewart, and medical students Alex Cumberworth and Joe Norris for their filming assistance
- Nick White and James Lewis at the Clinical Media Centre at the Royal Sussex County Hospital for their advice and help
- Daniel James for his extraordinary computer skills and patience in teaching me a few of them
- Ben Rony, John Tosh and Josh Lawson for their technical and/or video advice
- At Wiley, Elizabeth Paul for her copy-editing; David Gardner for his illustrations; Cathryn Gates and Karen Moore for helping get it all together
- And of course Martin Davies, publisher extraordinaire—whose support, guidance and company for lunch have been completely invaluable. A publisher of the highest order

Personal

- Aron, without whose patience, kindness and support during this project, it would never have got off the ground
- The parents what made me. And for all the encouragement and interest since then

Contents

List of Contributors, viii
Foreword by *John Black,*
President of the Royal College
***of Surgeons*, xi**
Preface, xii

General

1 Inguinal Hernia Repair, 1
Matt Stephenson and Stephen Whitehead
2 Split Skin Graft, 8
Matt Stephenson and George H C Evans
3 Femoral Hernia Repair, 13
Matt Stephenson and Paul Farrands
4 Incision and Drainage of Abscess, 20
Matt Stephenson and George H C Evans
5 Wedge Resection for Ingrown Toenail, 24
Matt Stephenson and Andrew Sandison
6 Paraumbilical and Umbilical Hernia
Repair, 28
Matt Stephenson and Stephen Whitehead
7 Appendicectomy, 34
Matt Stephenson and George H C Evans
8 Establishing a Pneumoperitoneum, 40
Matt Stephenson and Philip Ridings
9 Laparotomy, 44
Matt Stephenson and Don Manifold

Vascular

10 Long Saphenous Vein Stripping, 51
Matt Stephenson and Mike Brooks
11 Short Saphenous Vein Ligation, 57
Matt Stephenson and Mike Brooks
12 Abdominal Aortic Aneurysm Repair, 60
Matt Stephenson and Mike Brooks
13 Below Knee Amputation, 68
Matt Stephenson and Mike Brooks

14 Carotid Endarterectomy, 74
Matt Stephenson and Syed Wacquar Yusuf
15 Temporal Artery Biopsy, 82
Matt Stephenson and Utham R Shanker
16 Femorodistal Bypass, 85
Matt Stephenson and Karim El-Sakka
17 Brachiocephalic Fistula, 91
Matt Stephenson and Karim El-Sakka

Urology

18 Scrotal Exploration, 95
Matt Stephenson and Stephen Whitehead
19 Vasectomy, 99
Matt Stephenson and Vasileios Trompetas
20 Circumcision, 103
Matt Stephenson and Matthew Fletcher
21 Nephrectomy, 107
Matt Stephenson and Philip Thomas

Orthopaedics

22 Dynamic Hip Screw, 112
Matt Stephenson and Lisa Leonard
23 Hip Hemiarthroplasty, 121
Matt Stephenson and Lisa Leonard
24 Carpal Tunnel Decompression, 126
Matt Stephenson and Anand P Joshi

Upper Gastrointestinal

25 Gastrectomy, 130
Matt Stephenson and Peter C Hale
26 Splenectomy, 138
Matt Stephenson and Don Manifold
27 Gastrojejunostomy, 144
Matt Stephenson and Peter C Hale
28 Open Cholecystectomy, 148
Matt Stephenson and Peter C Hale
29 Thoracotomy, 155
Matt Stephenson and Don Manifold

Breast

30 Mastectomy, 160
Matt Stephenson and Elizabeth F Shah
31 Wide Local Excision, 166
Matt Stephenson and Elizabeth F Shah
32 Axillary Node Clearance, 171
Matt Stephenson and Elizabeth F Shah
33 Fibroadenoma, 178
Matt Stephenson and Elizabeth F Shah

Ear, Nose and Throat

34 Thyroidectomy, 181
Matt Stephenson and John S Weighill
35 Tracheostomy, 187
Matt Stephenson and John S Weighill

Colorectal

36 Haemorrhoidectomy, 191
Matt Stephenson and Peter J Webb
37 Colostomy and Other Stomas, 196
Matt Stephenson and Clare Byrne
38 Small Bowel Resection and
Anastomosis, 201
Matt Stephenson and Jeremy S Clark

39 Excision of Pilonidal Sinus, 206
Matt Stephenson and Stephen Whitehead
40 Right Hemicolectomy, 209
Matt Stephenson and Peter J Webb

Appendices

41 Surgical Instruments, 217
Matt Stephenson and Cheryl Funnell
42 Sutures, 227
Matt Stephenson and Cheryl Funnell
43 Patient Safety and the WHO Surgical
Checklist, 231
Matt Stephenson and Christopher M Butler
44 Theatre Etiquette, 237
Matt Stephenson and Ginny Bowbrick
45 How to Write the Operation Note, 241
Matt Stephenson and Petra Marsh
46 Consent, 246
Matt Stephenson

Index, 253

List of Contributors

Miss Ginny Bowbrick FRCS (Gen)
Consultant Vascular Surgeon
Medway NHS Foundation Trust
Medway Maritime Hospital
Windmill Road
Gillingham
Kent ME7 5NY

Mr Mike Brooks FRCS (Eng), FRCS (Gen)
Consultant Vascular Surgeon
Brighton and Sussex University Hospitals
NHS Trust Royal Sussex County Hospital
Eastern Road
Brighton BN2 5BE

Mr Christopher M Butler MS, FRCS
Consultant General Surgeon
Medway NHS Foundation Trust
Medway Maritime Hospital
Windmill Road
Gillingham
Kent ME7 5NY

Miss Clare Byrne FRCS
Consultant General and Colorectal Surgeon
Lewisham Healthcare NHS Trust
Lewisham High Street
London SE13 6LH

Mr Jeremy S Clark BSc, MSc, FRCS
Consultant Colorectal Surgeon
Brighton and Sussex University Hospitals
NHS Trust Royal Sussex County Hospital
Eastern Road
Brighton BN2 5BE

Mr Karim El-Sakka MD, FRCS
Consultant Vascular Surgeon
Brighton and Sussex University Hospitals
NHS Trust Royal Sussex County Hospital
Eastern Road
Brighton BN2 5BE

Mr George H C Evans MA, MChir, FRCS
Consultant General and Vascular Surgeon
East Sussex Hospitals NHS Trust
Eastbourne District General Hospital
Kings Drive
Eastbourne
East Sussex BN21 2UD

Mr Paul Farrands DM, FRCS
Consultant General and Colorectal
Surgeon
Brighton and Sussex University Hospitals
NHS Trust Royal Sussex County Hospital
Eastern Road
Brighton BN2 5BE

Mr Matthew Fletcher MS, FRCS
Consultant Urologist
Brighton and Sussex University Hospitals
NHS Trust Royal Sussex County Hospital
Eastern Road
Brighton BN2 5BE

Mrs Cheryl Funnell RGN
Lead Practitioner, General and Emergency
Team and Registered Nurse
East Sussex Hospitals NHS Trust
Conquest Hospital
The Ridge
St Leonards-on-Sea
East Sussex TN37 7RD

**Mr Peter C Hale MA, MS, FRCS
(Gen)**
Consultant General and Upper GI
Surgeon
Brighton and Sussex University Hospitals
NHS Trust Royal Sussex County Hospital
Eastern Road
Brighton BN2 5BE

Mr Richard Harvey MRCS
Vascular Surgery Teaching Fellow
Brighton and Sussex University Hospitals
NHS Trust Royal Sussex County Hospital
Eastern Road
Brighton BN2 5BE

**Mr Anand P Joshi Dip Ortho DNB
(Ortho), FRCS (T & O)**
Consultant Orthopaedic Surgeon
Medway NHS Foundation Trust
Medway Maritime Hospital
Windmill Road
Gillingham
Kent ME7 5NY

**Mrs Lisa Leonard BA, MSc, FRCS
(T&O)**
Consultant Orthopaedic Surgeon
Brighton and Sussex University Hospitals
NHS Trust Royal Sussex County Hospital
Eastern Road
Brighton BN2 5BE

**Mr Don Manifold MA, MS, FRCS
(Gen)**
Consultant General and Upper GI
Surgeon
Brighton and Sussex University Hospitals
NHS Trust Royal Sussex County Hospital
Eastern Road
Brighton BN2 5BE

Miss Petra Marsh BSc, MRCS
Surgical Specialist Registrar
South East Thames Rotation

Mr Philip Ridings BM, DM, FRCS
Consultant Surgeon
Brighton and Sussex University Hospitals
NHS Trust Royal Sussex County Hospital
Eastern Road
Brighton BN2 5BE

Mr Andrew Sandison FRCS
Consultant General and Vascular
Surgeon
East Sussex Hospitals NHS Trust
Eastbourne District General Hospital
Kings Drive
Eastbourne
East Sussex BN21 2UD

Miss Elizabeth F Shah MSc, FRCS
Consultant Oncoplastic Breast Surgeon
East Sussex Hospitals NHS Trust
Conquest Hospital
The Ridge
St Leonards-on-Sea
East Sussex TN37 7RD

Mr Utham R Shanker FRCS, FCEM
Consultant in Emergency Medicine
East Sussex Hospitals NHS Trust
Eastbourne District General Hospital
Kings Drive
Eastbourne
East Sussex BN21 2UD

Mr Philip Thomas FRCS
Consultant Urologist
Brighton and Sussex University Hospitals
NHS Trust Royal Sussex County Hospital
Eastern Road
Brighton BN2 5BE

Mr Vasileios Trompetas MSc, FRCS
Consultant General Surgeon
East Sussex Hospitals NHS Trust
Eastbourne District General Hospital

Kings Drive
Eastbourne
East Sussex BN21 2UD

Mr Peter J Webb MS, FRCS
Consultant General and Colorectal
Surgeon
Medway NHS Foundation Trust
Medway Maritime Hospital
Windmill Road
Gillingham
Kent ME7 5NY

Mr John S Weighill FRCS
Consultant ENT/Head and Neck Surgeon
Brighton and Sussex University Hospitals
NHS Trust Royal Sussex County Hospital
Eastern Road
Brighton BN2 5BE

Mr Stephen Whitehead MChir, FRCS
Consultant General Surgeon
East Sussex Hospitals NHS Trust
Conquest Hospital
The Ridge
St Leonards-on-Sea
East Sussex TN37 7RD

Mr Syed Wacquar Yusuf DM, FRCS
Consultant Vascular and Endovascular
Surgeon
Brighton and Sussex University Hospitals
NHS Trust Royal Sussex County Hospital
Eastern Road
Brighton BN2 5BE

Foreword

by John Black, President of the Royal College of Surgeons

One of the major advantages of the minimally invasive revolution of the last 25 years is that in procedures done that way no longer does the operating surgeon get the best, and often the only view of what is going on. Now everybody in the operating theatre sees exactly the same picture as the operator. Indeed many hospitals have facilities to transmit images to their education centre, or even anywhere else in the world. It is also easy to build up a comprehensive library of procedures, and several exist. There are also advantages to the trainer. One can feel more safely in charge of an operation when un-scrubbed watching the same monitor than when retracting for a trainee doing an open operation, particularly in an obese patient.

Unfortunately, many operations are not and never will be done endoscopically. This means that the trainee cannot become familiar with them beforehand in quite the same way as with a minimally invasive procedure. These are also the basic operations of surgery, the first that the trainee comes across and has to learn to do.

This book with its accompanying DVDs does its best to fill that gap. The common open operations of everyday surgical life that constitute the basic repertoire for all surgeons are presented here with a written commentary in practical vernacular style. It also allows access to a wide range of procedures, and even in the days before working time restrictions and other factors reducing clinical experience came into play it was never possible to have seen all the common operations.

The project is aimed at pre- and peri-MRCS surgical trainees and others at that level of experience, but others of far greater seniority will find it of interest. We haven't all seen everything!

John Black
President of the Royal College of Surgeons
March 2011

Preface

I hear and I forget
I see and I remember
I do and I understand
Confucius

Welcome to this, the first and only book and DVD resource showing real operations step-by-step in a manner not only helpful to the MRCS examinations, but to everyday practice. I set up this project, first because there was nothing else like it, but also because a commonly heard complaint from MRCS candidates is that they have to talk in their vivas, or now OSCEs, about operations they've never even seen. Even though the current exam doesn't have a specific operative surgery section as before, it still crops up for instance following the identification of a scar you've found whilst examining a patient. It's highly probable you'll have to describe an operation you've only ever read about—and that's not ideal. The examiner will be able to tell.

But this book and DVD are not just a resource to help you get through the exam, they're far more than that. *Learning to operate has never been so tough.* The European Working Time Directive has reduced the amount of time you spend in the hospital and consequently on time in theatre. It has also had a knock on effect on training time versus service time, with more time spent on nights or covering on call commitments. There may also be more doctors added to your rota, meaning more competition for space in theatre. What's more, the very practice of surgery is changing with the growth of minimally invasive surgery. It's quite possible your boss is only just learning how to do a laparoscopic right hemicolectomy him/herself, let alone let you loose on it. That could take up half of your precious list and all you've learnt is the art of keeping the camera still whilst yawning and shuffling your feet. Also, as data on operative outcomes (it started with cardiothoracics but is being rolled out further) become more available to the general public and litigation risks increase, with the enormous consequences this can have on service provision, the more your boss or department may feel they need to keep a tighter rein on the operating. With limited useful available time in theatre therefore, you have to make every moment count.

You want to get yourself to a high enough standard as quickly as possible so that if there's a hemiarthroplasty or right hemicolectomy on the list you get to do it, within reason, as early in your career as you can. The Royal College of Surgeons runs a course—*Training the Trainers*. One of its mantras is a four-stage teaching technique, essentially breaking down the advice to the trainer as:

1 Perform the procedure at a normal pace with the trainee watching without explanation, as you would normally do it
2 Perform the procedure at a pace to allow the trainee to see and understand each step with explanations as you go
3 Perform the procedure but have the trainee tell you what to do next
4 Let the trainee perform the procedure explaining all the steps to you

So if you've at least watched the procedure, maybe a handful of times from one of these videos, the first time you see it *in vivo* it won't be so unfamiliar, getting you a leg up on the learning curve that little bit earlier. In fact, potentially straight on to stage 3 or 4. Clearly nobody, hopefully, is going to stick rigidly to that mantra—otherwise it would mean if you have been in a 6-month job and only three open right hemicolectomies have come up (when you're not on nights/ annual leave/ study leave/ postnights enforced compensatory rest/ prenights enforced compensatory rest/ covering someone else/ on call) by these rules you wouldn't have even got your hands on one of them,

so it of course needs adaptability from the trainer. But your trainer is likely to be substantially more adaptable if you come to theatre preloaded with the knowledge. Proper Prior Planning Prevents Piss Poor Performance as they say.

You might also be interested to know that there are four stages of competence:

1 *Unconscious incompetence:* you really haven't the first idea how much you don't know/ can't do
2 *Conscious incompetence:* you begin to realise how little you know/ can do, and can't do it
3 *Conscious competence:* suddenly, you know stuff/ can do stuff and you know it
4 *Unconscious competence:* gradually, without you noticing, you know stuff/ can do stuff but you've known it for so long the novelty's worn off and it's second nature (this is often the reason for the phenomenon of the pant wetting stage of 'I don't know ANYTHING' just before an exam, followed by acing it).

Hopefully this book and DVD will catapult you out of any Stage 1ishness you have about you into stage 2 and, combined with actual operating, direct you into that wondrous, life-assuring, endorphin-releasing stage 3—you can do a splenectomy, and you know it.

But this is not just about exam revision, it's a vital resource for real life practice. I wish I'd seen this DVD before my first set of nights as a registrar.

Almost every operation here is performed (or occasionally supervised) by an experienced NHS consultant, who is an expert in their field (the only registrar led operations were the *Femoral Hernia*, *Incision and Drainage of Abscess* and *Appendicectomy* as these were in the middle of the night, and, let's face it, what are the chances of getting a consultant to do an abscess [the videos have however since been watched and endorsed by consultants]—I apologise in advance for my irritating radio voice, by the way). You will be shown a standard, safe way to perform each procedure. Yes of course Mr X does it this way and Prof Y does it another way, at Hospital Z. We're showing just one good way of doing it. There will be moments when you, or a colleague, watching these videos will vehemently criticise one particular technique shown because it's not the way you've seen it being done so far. This is the way with surgery—there is rarely just one way of doing it. Again, we show just one acceptable, safe, tried and tested way of doing it. We will also focus specifically on the operation, not the pathology—of that there is an abundance in other books.

Is this book evidence based? Well, no, not really. With the occasional exception, the aim has not been to present a set of evidence as to why something is best done a particular way. Usually no such evidence exists but here you will find the testimony of years of reflective consultant experience, hopefully that will suffice.

In the manner of so many previous inadequate authors I have elected to start this chapter with a quote from olden times from a much wiser man, mainly to disguise my own inadequate writing skills. I think Confucius was right, you can hear people describe something to you or read about it until you're sick of it, but until you see it with your own eyes, you just can't quite *appreciate* it. I remember the first time I saw Grey–Turners sign. It wasn't that I thought all the people who wrote medical textbooks were liars and scoundrels, it was just difficult to really, you know, imagine it. Then I saw it and haven't doubted it for a minute since. Until you see something with your own eyes your brain won't reach that crucial stage of belief, remembrance and understanding.

So what has been included? Well as you will already know, there isn't a definitive list of operations that the Royal College of Surgeons or the Joint Committee on Surgical Training have demanded we know. We have therefore combined all the available opinion about what comes up from the syllabus, other books on the subject, pooled experience of past MRCS candidates, common sense and to a certain pragmatic extent, just what could actually be filmed. We've tried to cover the most common operations you're likely to encounter on, for instance, a core surgical rotation. Of course there are so many more, but you have to stop somewhere, and 40 plus operations seemed reasonable . . .

Something you perhaps need to know about the videos themselves is just how difficult it is to produce a DVD like this.

You really can't imagine. For some time I was amazed at why no one else had tried it before, it gradually became clear why no one has. First, there was the clearance from the legal departments of the Trusts (more than one to increase the yield), ensure all the right paperwork was in order, from cycling proficiency test certificates to hepatitis B immunisations. Then to find the right pathology, in the right patient, who consented to being filmed (actually the easiest thing in the process, we owe our patients a huge amount. As it happens not one patient objected to being part of this process, and some of them participated extremely enthusiastically), with the right surgeon at the right time in the right theatre, with the right person and equipment (which works) available to film it: tricky. Some operations are easier to film than others for obvious reasons. These limitations mean it's simply not possible to get everything on film, so please forgive me, but I have tried.

I don't of course know quite what stage you're at. I'm fairly sure however that whether you're a medical student, Foundation Year 1, Core Surgical Trainee (the median audience aim for this book/DVD), Surgical Registrar, GP with a Specialist Interest in Surgery, Nurse, Operating Department Practitioner or hypochondriacal patient, this guide will start at a no nonsense all inclusive stage. But it won't leave you there. Each section isn't just a taster in its genre, in many cases it is an expert guide. Don't be put off by the level of detail in some chapters; the fact is, you can't half-learn an operation, you need a certain level of detail to really get to grips with it.

You will notice there's not much on laparoscopic surgery; that's partly because it doesn't play a huge part in MRCS or the early stages of surgical training. To begin with you want to learn how to do a 'proper' operation. Furthermore, the only video resources freely available up until now have concerned themselves almost solely with laparoscopic or other minimally invasive surgery (the availability of which exponentially increases with its rarity, complexity and operator ego). We hope to return to this growing area of surgery in a future edition.

As you will have astutely noticed, there is a book accompanying this DVD; you're currently reading it. Each chapter will closely mirror each chapter of the DVD. In each there is an introduction, a detailed explanation of each procedure running smoothly (which tends to quite closely follow what happens in the video) with video stills and other pertinent pictures and then sometimes a separate section discussing any particular points of interest or tips on difficult problems. Finally, each chapter has the key steps addressed in summary form. Obviously the operations aren't shown in real time—there wouldn't be space on three DVDs for that—so we've edited out or sped up the repetitive bits, or the bits we'd rather hadn't happened and wouldn't want you to see . . .

Lastly, I hope you enjoy it and I wish you the very best for your future career.

Matt Stephenson

A brief disclaimer: We don't put anywhere in the book or video that you should summon senior help if you need it. That's because it would become rather repetitive and it's just common sense. If you're out of your depth and need help—don't hesitate to ask.

1 Inguinal Hernia Repair

Matt Stephenson and Stephen Whitehead

> **Video** | **25 min 1 s**
> Stephen Whitehead, Consultant General Surgeon
> Conquest Hospital, St Leonards-on-Sea
> Filmed at Bexhill Hospital

Introduction

Inguinal hernia repairs are easy aren't they? Ermm... no, not really. Or at least not to begin with. The learning curve for an inguinal hernia is actually quite steep, probably because they can look so different every time you open the inguinal canal—it can be very frustrating. We've all been there. It never looks as clear as it does in the textbooks or atlases; it's almost as if the people who wrote those books had never seen one in real life. Like the appendicectomy, the inguinal hernia repair can be really quite difficult for the beginner, yet these two operations are still left to the most junior surgeons, often without supervision.

Nevertheless, take heart that everyone struggles to begin with and that once you've seen and done a few it will become second nature. Showing an inguinal hernia on video is actually rather tricky as the wound is quite small and the anatomy quite complex. Like many of the videos, you'll probably need to play it through a few times to take everything in. Here we show one whole operation all the way through and then in the *Inguinal Hernia Extras* video, a female inguinal hernia repair, an inguinoscrotal hernia and another indirect hernia so as to go over separating the cord and separating the sac—the bits everyone gets stuck on. Once you can do this, you've cracked it.

We are of course showing the Lichtenstein mesh repair—the most commonly used technique in the UK.

Procedure

With the patient **supine** and under **general** or **local** anaesthesia, **shave, prep** and **drape** the groin. Note the **bony landmarks** of the **anterior superior iliac spine (ASIS)** and the **pubic tubercle**. The **inguinal ligament** runs between these two. Your incision therefore needs to be a fingerbreadth or two **above and parallel** to the medial half to two-thirds of this.

Incise through **skin**, **Camper's fascia** and **Scarpa's fascia** (which is white and membranous) then through **fat**. It's likely

How to Operate: for MRCS Candidates and Surgical Trainees, First Edition. M. Stephenson. © 2011 John Wiley & Sons, Ltd. Published 2011 by John Wiley & Sons, Ltd.

you'll encounter a **chunky vein** running vertically in your wound—ligate and divide it if it's substantial enough, otherwise use diathermy. Keep incising down to **external oblique** maintaining **haemostasis** as you go. If the abdominal wall is quite thick, inserting a **Travers retractor** at this stage can be quite helpful.

You'll recognise the **aponeurosis** of external oblique by the fibrous strands running parallel to your wound. Once you've reached it, you need to decide the level at which you're going to open it. **Trace the fibres** down towards the pubic tubercle and look for where they **decussate**. That's what the **external ring** is, a triangular gap where the upper fibres plunge inferiorly to the lateral tip of the pubic tubercle and the lower fibres crisscross over and leap over to attach more medially. You can actually see this decussation and it marks the apex of the external ring where the hernia may be popping out.

So, make a **stab incision** in the line of the fibres at the level of the apex of the external ring. Take a small **clip** and clasp

the upper leaf and the same with the lower leaf. Using closed dissecting scissors bluntly **create a plane** below the external oblique in the line of the canal, thus separating off the cord or the **ilioinguinal nerve**, which may be sticking to it just below the surface. **Score** with the scissors inferomedially down to the external ring and the same superolaterally. With upward traction on the external oblique clips gently **dissect** beneath external oblique, superiorly and then inferiorly, thus **creating a plane** beneath it. Insert the Travers' retractors into this plane. **Congratulations**, you have now opened the inguinal canal. But, I'm sorry, you haven't fixed the patient yet; now comes the hard part. You look into the canal and unless you're very lucky, you just see a big bulging muscley, fatty, tissuey lump. What you're looking at is two things: the **cord** and the **sac** and they may be intimately entwined.

The first thing to do is separate the **cord (+/− sac)** from the **pubic tubercle**. Begin by **gently snipping**, with the tips of

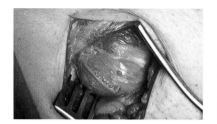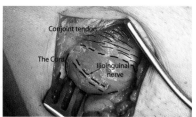

The bulging cord is shown outlined. Note the ilioinguinal nerve running over the front of it and the lower fibres of transversus abdominus which at their most inferior part form the conjoint tendon along with the internal oblique.

your scissors, any loose connective tissue that you can obviously see tethering the cord (+/− sac) down to the posterior wall of the inguinal canal. Next you need to **hook** the cord (+/− sac—that's getting boring, assume we mean potentially both for now) up **with your finger**. Insert your index finger into the inguinal canal with fingernail lying against the inside of the inguinal ligament with fingertip pointing to the pubic tubercle. Push your finger under the cord keeping your fingernail apposed to the pubic bone (there should be almost nothing between your fingernail and the bone—all the vessels etc. arching over the tubercle are staying with the cord—you don't want to leave them behind). Hook up the cord with your finger and **gently probe** with the fingertip until you **see it emerge** on the medial side of the cord. There is a knack to it and it comes with practise. It helps if you keep the axis of your finger horizontal, that is in line with the superior edge of the pubic bone, rather than pointing it upwards as you may just be pushing straight into a direct hernia.

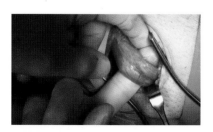

The cord has been hooked up by the index finger.

Once the cord is suspended over your hooked finger you need to work out **what's cord and what's sac**. To do this you first need to decide—is it an **indirect hernia** or a **direct hernia**? In an indirect hernia, the **whole cord is bulky** but it has a **relatively narrow base** (well, the same width as the rest of the cord) emerging from the deep ring and you can easily peel it off the posterior wall, which isn't bulging out. In a direct hernia however you will either feel a **thin cord** and behind it the **posterior wall is bulging out**, or, more likely, the whole cord seems to be coming from a **very wide base** stretching out over the whole of the back wall. This is because the sac emerging from the posterior wall has **fused** with the cord structures running past it. If this is the case, hook the cord inferoanteriorly and you'll see the posterior wall tethered up to the back of it. **Dissect** the connecting strands with scissors all the way back to the deep ring and the direct hernia bulge will fall back into its rightful place on the posterior wall and the cord will thin out. You may of course find **both**.

So, for the indirect hernia, the first part of this game is to find the **white edge** of the peritoneal sac. Everyone has their own favourite method of doing this. Here we show dissecting scissors gently peeling off the outer layers of the cord, all those cremasteric fibres, by firmly stroking the closed tips in the direction of the cord. Some people like to pinch the cord between finger and swab to firmly wipe off the outer layers and systematically

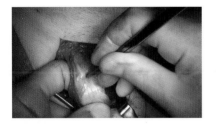

Dissection of the sac with the tips of the dissecting scissors.

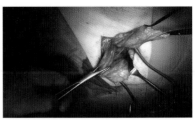

The sac has been dissected from the cord and is being retracted superiorly with clips whilst a Lanes retractor is retracting the cord inferiorly. A Langenbeck retractor exposes the posterior wall.

go from one edge transversely across to the other, thinning out the cord as they go. However you do it, you're looking for a white edge somewhere within the cord.

Once you see it, **get a clip** on it, get two if you can. Lift them up and gently **dissect all the adjacent tissue away** from the white edge, keeping close to the white edge, until the white edge gets bigger and bigger and more and more separate from the rest of the cord. If you're not sure where it's going, for example if you think it's going all the way down into the scrotum, you can **open it** and put your **finger inside**. Get the whole sac dissected out down to the level of the deep ring.

Twist the sac several times thus pushing any contents back into the abdomen and **transfix it** at the base with an absorbable suture such as 2–0 Vicryl. **Cut the stalk** of the sac first, not the stitch, that way you can check it's not bleeding before it dives back into the abdomen. If the deep ring has been widened by this intruder a **simple stitch** or two, **medially** and/or **laterally** to the ring will help.

Now, what if you find a direct hernia? This is much easier; you could just go straight to the mesh step but it's usually

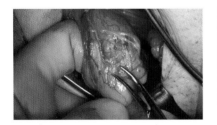

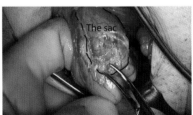

Identification of the sac.

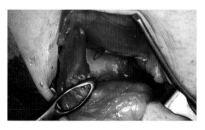

Gentle anteroinferior traction on the cord reveals the posterior wall—here it has been plicated.

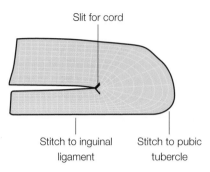

Slit for cord

Stitch to inguinal ligament

Stitch to pubic tubercle

The shape to cut the mesh into for a right-sided inguinal hernia. On the left obviously it's the mirror image.

easier to push the hernia back in with your finger, thus invaginating it, and then **plicate the posterior wall**. This stitch doesn't have much strength but it does make it easier to get the mesh down flat on the posterior wall. **Poke the hernia** back in with your index finger, this creates a **little ridge** of tissue (made of a bit of transversus abdominus and transversalis fascia) just above and below the tip of your finger in the medial part of the posterior wall—take a bite of the bottom ridge and then the top ridge and tie a knot (obviously taking care not to include your finger in the stitch). Keep stitching the bottom ridge to the top ridge until the hernia is essentially **inverted** and the back wall looks flat. Don't be overly ambitious with those stitches, trying for example to stitch strong muscle all the way down to inguinal ligament—this is unnecessary and just creates tension which is not what you want for wounds to heal. Also don't place the stitches too deep; don't forget that the **inferior epigastric vessels** aren't far behind.

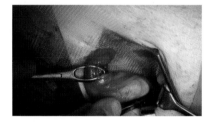

The mesh has been inserted with the upper and lower leaves wrapping around the base of the cord—the deep ring.

Now for the **mesh**. **Shape** it roughly before inserting it. The corner that will lie over the pubic tubercle can be rounded off. **Create a slit** so that you can wrap it round the cord—and at the apex of the slit create a **V-shape** so that the cord can fit through.

Stitch or **staple** the rounded corner to the tissue lying just over the **pubic tubercle**. It's very important that the mesh **overlaps the pubic tubercle**, and superiorly extends well beyond it, ideally to the **midline**—this is where the

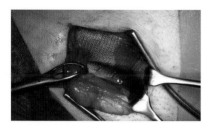

Completed mesh—note the inferior row of staples have been inserted onto the inside of the inguinal ligament.

hernia will recur if you don't. Hold the lower part of the mesh down so its lower edge is right over the inside of the **inguinal ligament**. Run a **continuous non-absorbable suture such as 2–0 Prolene**, suturing the two together; alternatively use staples. When you get to the deep ring, suture or staple the upper leaf to the lower leaf just lateral to the deep ring thus re-creating a new deep ring. Stitch the upper leaf down to the inguinal ligament. Not much else needs to be done laterally. Medially, you need to stitch the edge of the mesh down to the posterior wall, or staple it. **Stretch the mesh out** over the posterior wall so that it **isn't heaped up** or **too tight** and continue the suture or staples around the medial edge onto the superior edge. Take care to **avoid including a nerve** in your suture or staple.

If you've got this far and it's your first hernia—very well done to you. Now **close** up. Re-apply **clips** to the upper and lower edges of external oblique and run a **continuous absorbable suture such as 2–0 Vicryl** from lateral to medial or

medial to lateral, thus re-constructing the **external ring**. The **fascia** and **fat** can be closed with **continuous absorbable suture** and the **skin** with an **absorbable subcuticular suture**.

Notes

You'll see in the video that on finding an indirect hernia we don't do the usual twisting of the sac, transfixing and amputating it (which you can see in the *Inguinal Hernias Extras* video). This is because it's a sliding hernia as evidenced by the fat (and sometimes retroperitoneal structures like caecum) you can see in its wall. This is essentially a prolapse of the retroperitoneal tissues through the deep ring, rather than a processus vaginalis. If in doubt open the sac, if the lining has attached caecum inside, for instance, obviously you don't want to chop that off, so simply reduce it back to the abdomen.

In **women** (see *Inguinal Hernia Extras* video), inguinal hernia repairs are considerably easier. They have only rudimentary structures, principally the round ligament, passing through their inguinal canal—and this can be simply **ligated and divided**. The hernia can then be invaginated back into the abdominal cavity and the posterior wall plicated as for a direct inguinal hernia. You can then apply a piece of mesh without the usual slit to accommodate the cord, directly on to the posterior wall and stitch or staple it in.

In **inguinoscrotal** hernias (see *Inguinal Hernia Extras* video), the sac passes right through the canal into the scrotum where it's usually firmly adherent. **Don't try and dissect** the sac out of the scrotum—this will just result in lots of bleeding and is unnecessary. Instead, dissect out the sac in the usual way from the cord and **transect it**, leaving the distal part in the scrotum, undissected and **leave it open**. Any fluid that builds up in the residual sac will drain out of the hole, so don't close it or otherwise you're effectively giving the patient a hydrocoele. Deal with the proximal side in the same way as you would for any indirect hernia.

Summary

- The patient is **supine** and under **general** or **local anaesthetic**
- The correct groin is **shaved, prepped** and **draped**
- **Incise skin** above the medial half of the inguinal ligament
- Incise down to **external oblique**
- **Open** external oblique at the level of the external ring
- **Create a plane** beneath external oblique
- **Separate cord** +/− sac from the **pubic tubercle**
- Separate **cord from sac**
- **Transfix** and **amputate** indirect sacs
- **Plicate posterior wall** if bulging
- **Shape** and **insert** a mesh securing it, most importantly, medially
- **Close** the external oblique
- **Close** fascia then skin

2 Split Skin Graft

Matt Stephenson and George H C Evans

> **Video** | **7 min 13 s**
> George H C Evans, Consultant General and
> Vascular Surgeon
> Eastbourne District General Hospital, Eastbourne

Introduction

What's this one doing in a general surgical trainee's book/DVD I hear you ask. Well, you may have only worked in places with easy access to plastic surgeons but in many DGHs you won't have that advantage. Besides, this is an easy operation, which anyone can do, and having this skill significantly broadens your repertoire. It means you can boldly excise larger skin lesions where you can't get primary closure, encourage skin covering over laparostomy wounds and cover areas of skin loss following trauma—all without having to bother another team to get involved.

Probably the commonest indication for general surgeons is large skin lesions on the leg, particularly the shin, and especially in elderly folk who may have skin on their shin like parchment paper, and will just tear when you try to draw them together in primary closure.

Say you've biopsied a lesion on a patient's shin and it comes back as a melanoma of Breslow thickness 2.4 mm. You now need to go back and widely excise the scar, with 2 cm of clearance all the way around and down to deep fascia to reduce the risk of local recurrence. You're worried that you won't be able to get the edges together unless you are a bit more conservative with your excision. Hold your horses! Remember this is an oncological operation, much better to properly excise the lesion and margins. You may find this patient has been added to your day surgery list and whoever added her didn't consider how the skin edges would come together. If you don't think you'll be able to get the edges together without compromising on the margins, and therefore can't do an oncologically sound operation, don't be afraid to defer the operation. Find a time when the patient can put their feet up for 5 days postoperatively and there is time on the theatre list (they also need to usually stay at least one night even if they're young). If it

How to Operate: for MRCS Candidates and Surgical Trainees, First Edition. M. Stephenson. © 2011 John Wiley & Sons, Ltd.
Published 2011 by John Wiley & Sons, Ltd.

means a big hole on the leg which you can't close primarily so be it—this is where the split skin graft comes in.

Here, we'll use that example but the same principles apply wherever you're harvesting the skin from, or grafting it on to.

Procedure

With the patient under **general anaesthetic** (see Notes) and in an appropriate position given the location of the lesion to be excised (so supine if on the shin), **prep** the leg as usual and the harvest site just with **sterile water**. **Drape** the lesion and harvest site as appropriate.

Excise the lesion following **oncological principles;** don't be measly if this is proven to be, or highly suspicious for, cancer. Obtain **haemostasis** in the lesion bed but be sparing with the diathermy, the graft won't take on to a charcoaled bed, but neither will it onto a haematoma. Simple, prolonged pressure with a swab is often enough.

Set up your **dermatome**. The commonest one in use is the **air dermatome**, which is roughly the shape of one of those handheld windscreen squeegees. You

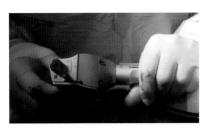

The dermatome is being prepared—the black dial on the side sets the depth of skin to harvest.

need to set two things. Firstly, choose the **width** of the blade (there are a variety of sizes to choose from) and put this into your dermatome. Secondly, there is a little switch where you can set the **depth** of skin to take. If the patient has very thin, aged and steroid-worn skin, take a thinner slice. If the skin is otherwise normal, take a thicker slice. On the handle there is a **safety switch** which needs to be flicked; once it has been, squeezing the handle gets it revving.

Usually the best place to **harvest** from is the **ipsilateral thigh**, either anterior or lateral. Get your assistant, if you have one, to **stretch** the skin of the donor site, either with their hands or the two small wooden boards usually provided on the set. The idea is to make the skin **taut** and **flat** so whatever makes this happen is fine. Drip some **sterile water** over the skin so the dermatome will glide smoothly. Press it down **fairly firmly** against the skin of the harvest site and then do **two things** at the same time: **press the lever** on the dermatome, getting it revving, and start **moving it forward** over the skin at a **slow steady pace** with **even** pressure across the area of contact. Move forward however far you think you'll need to harvest and then **lift** the dermatome off the skin, as soon as it's off the skin – let go of the lever. At this point don't do

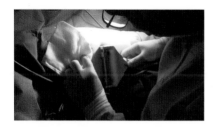

The dermatome in action.

anything – **pause** with the dermatome suspended a few millimetres above the skin. You need to check that the graft has separated off from the donor site; it often hangs on by a thread which can then rip and make a complete mess of your graft—cut the strand with a knife or scissors if necessary. **Flick the safety switch** of the dermatome disabling it.

Using two pairs of **non-toothed forceps** pick up the graft at two of its corners and lay it out on a moist surface on the scrub person's trolley. It always tries to **curl up** so carefully drag the edges out. Always remember which side is external

and which side is internal. It always tries to **curl inwards**, not outwards.

You now need to make lots of **holes** in it and **stretch** it out. You can't just lay it on as is, unfortunately. You need lots of holes in it to allow the usual fluid that builds up on the recipient wound to **drain out** and not collect under the graft, thus pushing it off. You need to **make it bigger** so that you can use a smaller patch of donor skin for a larger recipient site. You can easily have a recipient wound **three times bigger** than the donor site. Two options then to achieve this. You can use a **mesher**, which resembles a miniature old fashioned mangle. Place the graft on the clear plastic piece provided, fully stretched out. Insert the plastic piece into the mesher and wind the handle. It comes out looking like a mesh or a fishing net or similar. Alternatively, you can just make lots of **little fenestrations** with an 11 blade.

Check the recipient site looks dry and healthy. **Pick up the graft** with two pairs of forceps and carefully **lay it onto the wound**. It can be very fiddly

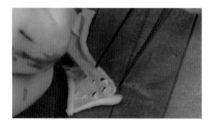

The graft is placed on a plastic surface and the edges unrolled. It is then fenestrated numerous times.

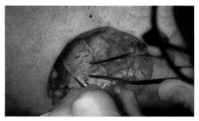

The graft being laid onto the wound.

because of the pleasure it takes in curling up and also in sticking to your forceps. **Persevere**. Don't lay it down the wrong way up.

Once it's on and the whole wound is covered, it may require some **shaping** of the graft to fit well. You then need to **fix it in place**. There are various options, one is a few interrupted **sutures** or even **staples**, say at each corner just anchoring to the adjacent skin edge. Alternatively you can use a **glue** like Dermabond around the edge. That graft needs to be **firmly pressed** against the donor site somehow. There are various options. First of all, use a **non-adhesive dressing** like Mepitel so the whole thing doesn't lift straight off when you take the dressings down (which would be highly embarrassing) and then a few layers of something like **gauze swabs/blue swabs/cotton wool** and then **wool and crepe**. **VAC dressings** work very well – they apply the pressure and remove any of the wound fluid that can push the graft off.

Whatever you've chosen it needs to stay on for **5 days** before inspection and the leg needs to be **strictly elevated** (less important if using a VAC) for that time. People vary as to how they like the donor site dressed. You can just use a clear waterproof dressing (like Opsite) some people use this but with **lignocaine soaked Kaltostat** applied on to the wound. Others use more elaborate methods, but as long as **air is kept out** of it, it should be relatively painless.

Notes

It can be done under **local anaesthetic** if there's good reason. You'll need to use quite a lot of dilute local, and it's a bit of a nuisance. Infiltrate as per normal for the lesion to be excised then mark out a rectangle on the harvest site (usually the anterior/ lateral thigh) with a marker pen and use a long slender epidural needle to infiltrate the skin of the harvest site.

The most important considerations about using a skin graft, other than the oncological principles mentioned above, is when it's **not** appropriate to use a split skin graft. The main contraindications are active **infection** at the recipient site (treat it first with antibiotics etc.), **insufficient blood flow**, either arterial or venous (treat these first as appropriate) and the lack of a **healthy bed** to graft on to. It won't take on bone or cartilage for instance; here you will need more elaborate flaps or full-thickness skin grafts. A laparostomy wound needs to have fully granulated first, for instance.

Summary

- With the patient under **general anaesthetic**, **prep** and **drape** the lesion excision/ recipient site and the donor site
- **Excise** the lesion/ prepare the recipient site
- Set up the **dermatome** choosing **width** and **depth**
- **Take the skin graft** using firm even pressure
- **Fenestrate** and **stretch** out the graft by manual means or mesher
- **Place on** recipient site and **shape**
- **Fix** in position with sutures/ staples/ glue
- **Press on firmly** with non-adhesive dressing then other dressings
- **Dress** donor site with waterproof/ airproof dressing
- **Elevate** for 5 days

3 Femoral Hernia Repair

Matt Stephenson and Paul Farrands

> **Video** | **14 min 27 s**
> Matt Stephenson, Surgical Registrar
> Royal Sussex County Hospital, Brighton

Introduction

Femoral hernias are far less common than inguinal hernias. If you've only seen or done the latter so far, you might be worrying how much more mysterious and complex a femoral hernia could possibly be. The good news is—they're actually easier. Whereas it might take 20 inguinal hernia operations to be able to competently do anything the inguinal canal cares to throw at you, once you've done a femoral hernia, you've done them all.

OK so that's not strictly true—because there are four main approaches to fixing them but it's certainly true of each of them. The **Lockwood** approach can be used for elective femoral hernias, where there's no clinical concern that the patient has incarcerated bowel. The three other approaches are the **McEvedy**, **Lothiessen** and standard **midline**. These can be used for femoral hernias where there is concern for bowel viability. A laparotomy, Lothiessen and McEvedy all fix the hernia in exactly the same way (i.e. from the inside of the canal, rather than the outside as in a Lockwood repair); they only differ in how you get though the abdominal wall in order to get to the inside of the femoral canal. It's largely a matter of personal preference which one you choose but the McEvedy is our preferred approach.

We'll describe each of them here but have filmed the modified McEvedy approach as this is the one to get you out of trouble in the middle of the night when you're worried about incarcerated bowel.

The modified McEvedy

With the patient **supine** under **general anaesthetic** and the correct groin and lower quadrant **shaved** and **prepped**, locate the **bony landmarks** of the **pubic tubercle and anterior superior iliac spine (ASIS)** to orientate yourself. The femoral hernia is found **below and lateral** to the pubic tubercle. Make a **transverse** incision in the right lower quadrant. It is

How to Operate: for MRCS Candidates and Surgical Trainees, First Edition. M. Stephenson. © 2011 John Wiley & Sons, Ltd.
Published 2011 by John Wiley & Sons, Ltd.

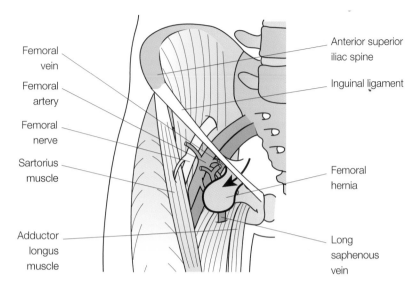

Femoral vein	Anterior superior iliac spine
Femoral artery	Inguinal ligament
Femoral nerve	
Sartorius muscle	Femoral hernia
Adductor longus muscle	Long saphenous vein

The femoral hernia and its relations.

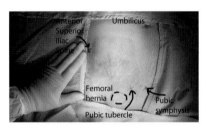

The relevant landmarks in this patient's right lower quadrant and groin.

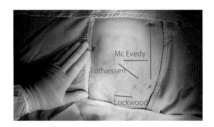

The four approaches for a femoral hernia.

placed about one-third of the way from pubic symphysis to umbilicus, from the midline to about the midclavicular line. (NB McEvedy initially described a vertical incision over the lateral lower edge of rectus but that results in an ugly, painful scar—this way, you get the same access but less ugliness and pain).

Deepen the incision through **superficial fascia** and **fat** down to the rectus sheath. Now **divide the rectus sheath** more or less **vertically** at its **edge** where it merges with external oblique. Once through the anterior rectus sheath, you can easily **retract** the **rectus abdominus medially** with Langenbeck retractors. Immediately behind this is peritoneum, or if you've gone in a bit too high up you'll encounter posterior rectus sheath.

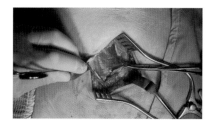

Rectus sheath has been incised along its length and the edges are held apart with clips, revealing the rectus abdominus within.

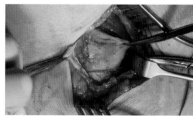

The rectus abdominus has been retracted medially exposing peritoneum.

Divide the peritoneum and you're in the abdomen. Retract the lower edge of the wound and **feel** down to the internal opening of the femoral canal—you're right over it with this incision (you can often feel it better than you can see it). Here you'll find the hernial contents, which may be omentum or bowel, have been drawn into the internal orifice. Between finger and thumb very gently **try to manipulate** the herniated contents back into the abdomen, **pressure externally** over the palpable groin lump can help. Sometimes you can't reduce it this way, so, if you can't, **pick up the peritoneum** with a clip and **dissect** (usually with your fingers is enough) in the **extraperitoneal plane** down to the neck of the femoral hernia and gently try to **reduce** the peritoneal sac. You probably won't be able to reduce the whole sac as it forms adhesions in the groin but you should be able to reduce the contents in this way. If you can't, try a third manoeuvre—dissect under the skin through the subcutaneous fat down to below the inguinal ligament

(the skin is this stretchy, especially in elderly ladies that get femoral hernias). You can then dissect out the sac where it emerges from the femoral canal (like you would do in a Lockwood approach). You can open it and by a combination of pushing from here and pulling from inside, the contents will reduce. Bowel is always reducible, omentum however often forms adhesions with the inside of the sac rendering it very difficult to reduce, and if you can it just bleeds in the sac which you can't do much about. It's better to just amputate off this troublesome omentum if it doesn't come easily.

Once reduced, **inspect** it for **viability**. Necrotic or suspect omentum is just amputated. **Necrotic** or **perforated bowel** will obviously need to be **resected** and two healthy ends anastomosed. Often the bowel just looks **bruised** and **distorted;** if so, **wrap** this in a **swab** soaked in warm saline and put it back in the abdomen to warm up and **re-inspect** after a few minutes. If the bowel surface

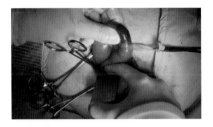

The small bowel has been delivered and inspection reveals a Richter's hernia with only a bruised bowel.

now looks **shiny**, if it's **peristalsing**, and if there's a **palpable pulsation** in the mesentery you won't need to resect it, but have a low threshold for resection otherwise.

Now to **repair** the femoral canal. If you couldn't reduce the sac from the canal then there will still be a plug of peritoneum stopping you from repairing it. Go back to the extraperitoneal space; as long as you're happy that the sac is empty, **cut straight across it** with diathermy thus leaving the fundus of the sac separated off to remain forever in the canal. You can then clearly see the femoral canal and its

borders (**anteriorly—inguinal ligament, medially—lacunar ligament, posteriorly—pectineal ligament, laterally—femoral vein)**. From the inside, stitch the **pectineal ligament posteriorly** to the **inguinal ligament anteriorly** with two or three non-absorbable stitches (or a mesh, as in the Lockwood approach, but don't use mesh if bowel was incarcerated).

Close the peritoneum with absorbable sutures and infiltrate some **local anaesthetic** into the rectus sheath and skin. Close the **anterior rectus sheath** with polydioxanone suture (PDS) or similar and **skin** with a subcuticular stitch.

Lothiessen

NB This approach is not particularly popular—because it means going in through the inguinal canal—and why would you choose to do this when the inguinal canal is hardly reputed for its robustness? And you're about to weaken it even further by cutting right through the posterior wall, which you're then going

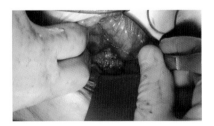

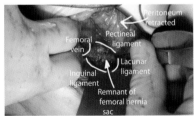

You are looking down at the internal orifice of the femoral canal which is still occupied by a remnant of sac filled with omentum. This is in the extraperitoneal plane, you can see the peritoneum has been reflected upwards.

to need to repair on the way back out. It may have an arguable role in situations where you're not sure preoperatively whether the groin hernia is inguinal or femoral or even if they have both.

With the patient **supine** under **general anaesthetic** and the right groin and lower quadrant **shaved** and **prepped**, proceed as in the inguinal hernia chapter (Chapter 1) until you've entered the inguinal canal. Then divide the posterior wall of the inguinal canal with diathermy looking out for the peritoneum, which you open with scissors between two clips. You've now entered the peritoneal cavity. Use your assistant to retract the lower edge of the wound, thus exposing the internal orifice of the femoral canal. Then proceed as with the McEvedy repair. When closing up you need to be meticulous about your repair of the posterior wall of the inguinal canal.

Midline laparotomy

Proceed with the usual opening of the abdominal wall and then continue as described in the McEvedy section. The advantages to doing it this way is, if you're inexperienced, a midline laparotomy is the easiest approach—you just go straight through the midline. It also means you can extend up and do a full laparotomy if there was some preoperative equivocality (e.g. a patient with bowel obstruction but a pre-existant non-tender femoral hernia, which may or may not be the cause). The disadvantages are the ugliness of a midline scar cutting though all of Langer's lines, and that from the midline you don't enter directly over the inside of the femoral canal.

Lockwood approach

With the patient **supine** under **general anaesthetic** or spinal, **shave** and **prep** the appropriate groin and abdomen. Locate the **bony landmarks** of the **pubic tubercle and ASIS** to orientate yourself. The femoral hernia is found **below and lateral** to the pubic tubercle.

Make a roughly **transverse incision** in a skin crease directly overlying the lump. Using diathermy (or a knife) carefully make your way through **superficial fascia** and **subcutaneous fat** looking out for the **hernia sac**, which has that somewhat glistening appearance of peritoneum. Insert a **self-retaining retractor** (such as a Travers'). Using scissors carefully **dissect** around **the hernia sac** separating off the adjacent tissues which often become adherent to it. Gently try to curl your finger around the neck of the sac and by a mixture of sharp and blunt dissection **free up the entire sac up to its neck**. The neck is the opening of the femoral canal; this is a small space, the boundaries of which are: **anteriorly— inguinal ligament**, **medially—lacunar ligament**, **posteriorly—pectineal ligament**, **laterally—femoral vein** (a femoral hernia therefore pokes out initially directly down to the floor, but often then curves anteriorly and can even wrap upwards around the inguinal ligament if large enough).

With the sac dissected out up to the neck, place two clips on it and using scissors **open the sac** to inspect the contents. This is almost always just fatty omentum and can be pushed back into the abdomen (this is sometimes the hardest bit to do and you'll realise why once you've got it back in—that canal can often barely take the tip of your little finger and the contents of the sac is much larger (imagine trying to resect bowel through it)). If you are struggling to reduce the contents, either **amputate the contents** of the sac by tying it off and ligating it, or, very gently with the tip of your little finger poked into the tight opening, **push anteriorly**, therefore stretching the inguinal ligament a millimetre or so (out of the four sides of the opening—this is the safest place to do this manoeuvre—obviously there's nothing you can do about the femoral vein which is compressible anyway, the lacunar ligament is said to contain an accessory branch of the obturator artery in 50% of cases, and that would be a nuisance, and the pectineal ligament is firmly stuck onto the bony pectineal line). Then **close the sac** with absorbable suture such as 2–0 Vicryl and return this to the abdomen too (it may be necessary to amputate most of this too if it won't go back in).

Next **close the femoral canal**. There are two options: **direct suture** using two or three non-absorbable interrupted sutures (e.g. 2–0 prolene) or **mesh**. In the former, stitch the pectineal ligament posteriorly to the inguinal ligament anteriorly (the problem can occasionally be if the femoral canal is quite large, there can be a lot of tension on this stitch as the pectineal ligament and inguinal ligament are fairly immobile and don't pull together). In the mesh repair, roll a square of polypropylene mesh diagonally and then fold this over on itself, making a sort of cigar-shaped plug. Push the plug up into the canal and stitch one limb to the pectineal ligament and the other to the inguinal ligament.

Close with one layer of continuous absorbable suture to fat/ fascia and absorbable subcutaneous continuous suture to skin and infiltrate with **local anaesthetic**.

Notes

You may have noticed that in the non-Lockwood approaches for incarcerated hernia, we've described opening the peritoneum at the earliest opportunity whereas many books talk about staying extraperitoneal and then opening the sac later. You can do this but it makes sense to try and assess and rescue the bowel as soon as you can, you're going to need to open the peritoneum at some stage anyway and if the bowel is easily reducible intraperitoneally it saves you some time. Often, however, it is not and you do then need to dissect in the extra-peritoneal plane.

Summary (modified McEvedy)

- The patient is **supine** under **general anaesthetic**
- The groin and abdomen is **shaved, prepped** and **draped**
- Make a **transverse incision** in the lower quadrant
- **Incise** the rectus sheath **vertically**
- **Retract** rectus abdominus **medially**
- Open **peritoneum**
- Try to **reduce contents intraperitoneally**
- If necessary try to **reduce extra-peritoneally**
- **Inspect contents** and assess viability
- **Divide neck** of sac if irreducible
- **Repair defect**, stitching pectineal ligament to inguinal ligament
- **Reassess** any bowel
- **Close peritoneum** with absorbable sutures
- **Close rectus sheath** with PDS
- Infiltrate **local anaesthetic**
- **Close skin** with absorbable continuous subcuticular suture

4 Incision and Drainage of Abscess

Matt Stephenson and George H C Evans

> **Video** | **4 min 45 s**
> Matt Stephenson, Surgical Registrar
> Royal Sussex County Hospital, Brighton

Introduction

This is the most basic and commonest operation you're likely to encounter on the emergency list. Nobody will ever teach you how to do one. It will be a given that you will naturally know. Fortunately there isn't much to it, but there are some important issues to consider to reduce the risk of an **early recurrence** (commoner in the less experienced surgeon), **minimise** the amount of tissue trauma and consequent **healing time**, and use **antibiotics** rationally.

Abscesses can occur almost anywhere in the body; here of course we talk about **superficial abscesses**, which are common in the **perianal, sacrococcygeal** (see *Excision of Pilonidal Sinus* Chapter 39) and buttock areas but also in the **axillae** and **groins, breasts** and **diabetic feet**. The principles are all similar wherever they are; make an incision **large enough** to drain the pus and **leave it open** to make sure it won't close up before the cavity does. Abscesses are therefore **never closed primarily**.

Location-specific differences are occasionally significant. Regarding perianal abscesses—these can arise either from the **anal glands**, in which case there is a risk of developing a fistula-in-ano, or from the **skin** of the buttock, in which case there is no risk of developing a fistula-in-ano. Taking a microbiological swab of the pus will help distinguish between the two as the former will grow **coliforms** and the latter will grow **skin bugs**. It's also

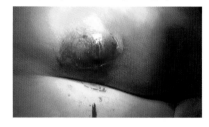

A right buttock abscess.

How to Operate: for MRCS Candidates and Surgical Trainees, First Edition. M. Stephenson. © 2011 John Wiley & Sons, Ltd. Published 2011 by John Wiley & Sons, Ltd.

sensible to do a full **examination under anaesthetic** (EUA) in these patients to feel digitally above the sphincter for **supralevator induration**, suggestive of deep ischio-rectal sepsis, and also to examine the rectal mucosa with a sigmoidoscope, mainly to check they don't have associated **proctitis**.

Regarding diabetic foot abscesses, these are often **not clinically obvious** and the only clue may be a discharging sinus. If there is **deep infection** in the foot, these need to be **urgently** drained before the infection rapidly spreads up the leg. Again open these widely, don't be afraid to debride all devitalised tissue just because you think you're being over destructive—the fact is it will never heal if necrotic tissue remains.

Depending on their size and location, some abscesses can be drained under **local anaesthetic**. These need to be superficial with no concern about deep extension; perianal abscesses are **never suitable** for local drainage therefore. Infected sebaceous cysts on the back of the neck often extend deeply. Local anaesthetic doesn't work well in areas of cellulitis, and, even if it does, there's a temptation to compromise on really curetting out the cavity properly as it will probably still hurt. Nevertheless, if it seems suitable you can save the patient from being admitted and undergoing a general anaesthetic.

Sometimes, by the time the patient is due to go down to theatre the abscess has **already burst**. Be cautious about cancelling them because of this—usually the pinhole that the pus leaks from quickly closes up again and the pus once again collects in the cavity. Generally speaking, there needs to be a generous hole to prevent repeat abscess formation and chronic sepsis.

It's contentious whether it's wasting the microbiology department's time by sending a pus swab of every single pedestrian abscess you drain—what difference does it make to the patient's management in an otherwise completely well patient with an uncompli-cated abscess?

Procedure

With the patient under **general anaes-thetic** (or **awake**) and in an appropriate position given the location of the abscess (always lithotomy for perianal abscesses), **prep** and **drape** the area. If you can avoid having to position the patient prone and doing it on their side, you'll become **popular** with the anaesthetist and the theatre staff as **positioning prone is more awkward**. If you're doing this under local anaesthetic, there isn't much point in injecting the local directly into the abscess or even the red skin overlying it—it won't work because of the **acidic** nature of the tissue and because the red **hyperaemic** skin carries the local away quickly. Instead inject the local in a **circle** all around the abscess forming a **field block**.

Usually, it is obvious where the centre of the abscess is because it's pointing to the skin with overlying **redness**, **fluctuance** or **induration**. If in doubt introduce a large bore **white needle** mounted on a syringe and suck where you think the pus is. If no pus is aspirated, try different places and eventually, once you strike gold, you'll know where to make the incision.

Make a **linear incision** over the abscess and insert a **microbiology swab** into the cavity (taking care to avoid the skin edges on the way in—you want a pus swab not a skin scraping). **Feel the satisfaction** as all the **pus drains away** into your kidney dish. Initially, just make the hole big enough to fit your finger into, **feel** around in the cavity digitally and **break down** any **loculations** of the abscess, feeling where the cavity seems to be going. Sometimes it extends off in a direction you weren't anticipating and having made a small incision to begin with you can now extend it over the cavity, minimising any unnecessary incision length. Ideally, you don't want to have too much cavity being covered by skin but this would sometimes mean having to have really huge incisions for relatively shallow cavities. Consider inserting a **corrugated drain** (such as a **Yates** drain) into such cavity extensions. This can work well for deep ischiorectal abscesses too. Some people make cruciate incisions in the skin if it is an expansive abscess. It's better to simply make the incision over where the cavity is, and if this happens to be in a cruciate shape so be it. Usually, however, a linear incision held open with packs is enough.

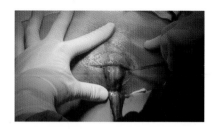

A linear incision is made over the abscess releasing a satisfying flow of pus.

If the skin edges look necrotic—excise them too.

Once you've made the wound large enough, use a **Volkmann spoon** to **curette** out the lining. This is because the fatty lining of the abscess cavity will be necrosing as the abscess is enlarging so you want to shred this out, but also in the case of some chronic abscesses you see a slimy layer of granulation tissue, which isn't the good kind of healthy granulation tissue essential to healing up these cavities, this needs to be scraped off first.

You'll then find it's probably **bleeding** quite a lot. **Irrigate** the whole cavity with some **normal saline** by **squirting** it with a 50 ml syringe **under pressure** into the cavity (protecting your eyes and all around you with your other hand), some people also use **hydrogen peroxide**. If there's profuse bleeding from a skin edge then **diathermy** is probably sensible to stop it, but usually it's just **oozing generally** from the cavity. You can't diathermy the whole cavity lining, this is a job for the **haemostatic pack**. Poke a gauze swab into the cavity and wait a while. The oozing always stops. Replace the gauze

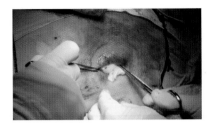
An Aquacel pack has been inserted.

swab with a haemostatic packing material such as **Aquacel** or **Kaltostat** and leave this in. Cover with **blue gauze** and a dry dressing like **Mefix**. The pack should be removed in **24** to **48** hours and replaced and the patient should be reviewed every couple of days by his practice nurse for dressing changes until the cavity has closed up.

Summary

- With the patient under **general anaesthetic, prep** and **drape** the area
- **Incise** directly over the abscess
- **Drain** away the pus after taking a **microbiology** swab
- **Break down** the **loculations** with a finger
- **Extend** the wound as necessary
- **Curette** the lining
- **Irrigate**
- **Haemostase**
- **Insert** a pack
- **Dry dressings**

5 Wedge Resection for Ingrown Toenail

Matt Stephenson and Andrew Sandison

> **Video** | **6 min 8 s**
> Andrew Sandison, Consultant General and Vascular Surgeon
> Eastbourne District General Hospital, Eastbourne
> Filmed at Bexhill Hospital

Introduction

Ingrown toenails are agony. Postoperative recovery after surgery for an ingrown toenail can be agony too, so the procedure you do for the patient has to work first time. Recurrences after ingrown toenail surgery can be disappointingly high if not done radically enough. Like so many procedures, there seem to be so many ways of doing it. We've shown this one because of its simplicity, low recurrence rate, rapid healing and good cosmetic result (this patient has already had a wedge excision on the other side of his hallux using this technique—note how well it's healed).

In the following procedure, we'll describe an ingrown toenail on the lateral side of the hallux as in the video; obviously it's the same principle on the medial side, and if you're doing both sides, just do both sides.

Procedure

In addition to your usual scrubbing, **eye protection** is particularly important as getting phenol in your eyes is a disaster. With the patient **supine** and **chatting** to a nurse (or unusually, as in the case of our needle phobic patient, under general anaesthetic), **prep** the foot including in between the toes, and **drape** around the forefoot. Inject a **ring block** at the base of the toe—about 3 ml of **0.5% plain bupivocaine** on each side of the toe. Wait for anaesthesia and test with toothed forceps. **Squeeze** the toe with your fingers and thumb and with the other hand wrap a **tourniquet** around the base of the toe to reduce bleeding.

You now need to take out your **wedge of tissue** and that includes the lateral edge of the nail and also the skin it's

---

How to Operate: for MRCS Candidates and Surgical Trainees, First Edition. M. Stephenson. © 2011 John Wiley & Sons, Ltd.
Published 2011 by John Wiley & Sons, Ltd.

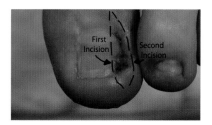

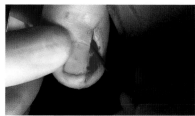

The two incisions necessary to excise the wedge.

Incising the nail matrix.

embedded in, which is usually infected or granulating. This is accomplished essentially by **two incisions**. The **first** is made over the **dorsal surface** by incising in a straight line (best done with a broad 10 blade), right through the nail and the skin proximal and distal to it; you may only need to excise the lateral 3 or 4 mm of nail. Make sure you use your finger against their toenail to stop the blade from slipping too deeply. The **second** incision is at an approximately **30–45 degree** angle to the last, around the side of the toe so that it meets with the first one—thus giving you a wedge of tissue. You can now **pull the wedge** of tissue out with a clip or **forceps**.

These incisions need to be **quite deep**, that is taking out quite a deep wedge—in fact almost down to **bone**. Nevertheless, you need to just check that you haven't left any nail matrix behind so peer into the cavity (nail matrix is **white** and **quite shiny)**; **excise** anything that's left with a narrower blade like an 11. So you have mechanically destroyed the nail matrix but there may be residual patches you've missed, so a sensible back up step is

to ablate the corner of the nail matrix **chemically** with **phenol**.

First, you need to **protect the skin** from the phenol as you obviously don't want to destroy that too. Take a Jelonet dressing and scrape off the **petroleum jelly** substance with a blunt instrument or wipe it directly onto the neighbouring skin around the cavity. Wipe this **liberally** over everything near the nail matrix that isn't the nail matrix. It will protect it from the phenol. Put a **cotton bud tip** into the **80% phenol** solution and stick it into the depths of the cavity. Leave it there for **3 minutes**, occasionally **twisting** it to ensure an even spread and then wash off with liberal amounts of **industrial**

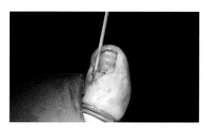

The tip of the cotton bud is soaked in 80% phenol solution.

methylated spirit, also useful for cleaning off the jelly. **Dry** it.

To close, two **steristrips** will suffice, the edges come together surprisingly easily. Just make sure they **don't completely encircle** the toe. Apply a little **non-adhesive dressing** over the wound itself, like the Jelonet you opened earlier. Then apply **blue gauze** circumferentially—not too tight but reasonably firmly—**remove the tourniquet** and make sure you can see the toe is **pinking up** through the hole in the end of the bandage. Put on a **crepe bandage** to hold it round the ankle to stop it falling off. Make sure the patient keeps the foot **elevated** for a good 24 hours, has plenty of **analgesia** and an appointment to see the **practice nurse** in 48 hours, who can downscale the dressings.

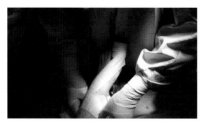

Blue gauze and crepe bandage.

Notes

There are two other options for ingrown toenails:

1 **Simple avulsion** of the nail—usually most appropriate in A and E when the patient comes in with frank infection around the nail. All that's needed is a ring block and to slide one jaw of an artery forceps under the nail, grasp the nail with the forceps and remove it by twisting the nail off—it will grow back but at least removing this 'foreign body' will let things settle down.

2 **Zadek's procedure**—for really recurrent, persistent nails where the patient is happy to accept the cosmetic implication that there'll be no nail ever there afterwards. In this operation, rather than removing a wedge of tissue, you make a diagonal incision from each corner of the nail and lift up the skin proximal to the nail, which you then avulse. Lifting up the flap of skin in skin hooks reveals all the nail matrix which you can then excise and ablate in the same way as in the procedure we're describing here. The skin flap can then be sutured back down on each side.

Summary

- Put on your **eye protection** before scrubbing
- Inject a **ring block**
- **Prep** and **drape** the foot
- Apply **tourniquet**
- Make first incision as described
- Make second incision as described, thus forming a wedge of nail and skin
- **Remove wedge** with forceps
- Remove any additional **macroscopic nail matrix**

- Apply **protective jelly** to adjacent skin
- Put in 80% **phenol** soaked cotton bud tip **for 3 minutes**
- **Irrigate** off with **industrialised methylated spirits**
- **Dry**
- Apply non-constricting **steristrips**

- Apply **non-adhesive dressing** and **blue gauze**
- **Release** the tourniquet
- **Crepe** bandage
- **Check the toe is pink**
- Advise **elevation, elevation, elevation** and prescribe **analgesia**

6 Paraumbilical and Umbilical Hernia Repair

Matt Stephenson and Stephen Whitehead

Video | 18 min 25 s
Stephen Whitehead, Consultant General Surgeon
Conquest Hospital, Hastings
Filmed at Bexhill Hospital

Introduction

This is a satisfying operation, and it's easy to learn! You can convert an ugly looking, often discoloured bulge on the abdominal wall into a nice flat contour with a normal looking umbilicus (usually). It's one of the bread and butter operations of the day case list but will also crop up on call as an emergency, so learn it first electively if you can.

There's not much difference between the surgical management of **umbilical** and **paraumbilical hernias**. The anatomical difference between them lies in the fact that in a paraumbilical hernia, the sac protrudes through the linea alba adjacent to the cicatrix (see later), but in the umbilical hernia the sac protrudes through the cicatrix itself. You can deal with this surgically in a very similar way. The defect is usually slightly smaller in the umbilical hernia. They have characteristic differences on examination: the paraumbilical hernia gives a crescentic skin fold whereas the umbilical hernia gives a complete circle of a skin fold. Umbilical hernias are particularly common in infants, especially of African descent, and should generally be left alone unless they haven't resolved by the age of 3 years.

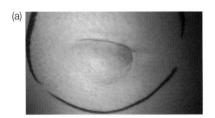 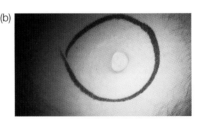

(a) Paraumbilical; (b) umbilical.

How to Operate: for MRCS Candidates and Surgical Trainees, First Edition. M. Stephenson. © 2011 John Wiley & Sons, Ltd.
Published 2011 by John Wiley & Sons, Ltd.

Procedure

It helps to **mark the hernia** preoperatively with the patient standing with a permanent marker by drawing a circle/ovoid shape around the maximum limit of the lump (when the patient is under general anaesthetic and muscle relaxation, the hernia sometimes spontaneously reduces and it helps to remember exactly where it comes out and the extent of it). With the patient **supine** and under **general anaesthesia**, **shave, prep** and **drape** the abdomen around the umbilical hernia.

Make a **slightly curved incision**. If it's a small hernia, make it in the umbilical skin fold for the best cosmetic result. Mark your incision with a skin marker first of all—it's very difficult to make a nice symmetrical incision if you don't, particularly because the umbilical skin can be so stretchy. Using a small blade helps with this as it goes round a small radius curve easier than a large one. This can be either directly **over the lump**, or it can be made a little inferior to the **crescentic skin fold** that typifies paraumbilical hernias. As soon as you've gone **through the skin**, **stop** and **reassess**. As paraumbilical hernias enlarge, the number of planes between skin and peritoneal sac reduces until in very large, chronic paraumbilical hernias, basically **skin = sac**. In the emergency setting therefore, remember incarcerated bowel maybe 2 mm below the surface. Take your **Allis forceps** and gently apply them to the **superior skin edge** of your wound—

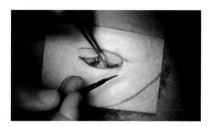

The curved incision, the forceps start to lift the flap superiorly.

trying if you can to pinch the subcutaneous tissue rather than the actual external skin surface. Ask your assistant to **lift them up** towards the ceiling. With a swab in your non-dominant hand press down on the lower skin edge creating tension between the superior skin edge and what lies beneath. Using scissors gently **dissect down** between the two skin edges until you find that characteristic white **peritoneal sac;** it's usually very close under the skin.

Continue to **dissect close to the sac** using a mixture of scissors and blunt dissection, keeping **traction** on the skin edges, follow the sac down to its **neck**, where it meets the **fascia** (that tough looking white fibrous layer—essentially where the rectus sheaths from each side meet at the linea alba). Then work your way around the neck of the sac, making sure you can see the **junction of sac–fascia** all the way around the top half of the neck. Swap places with your assistant and ask him/her to reapply the Allis forceps to the **inferior skin edge** and repeat the process of dissecting out the sac down to the fascia. Beware that the plane between skin and sac can be **perilously close** and it's easy to **'button hole'** the skin if you're not careful. Also, you'll find the dissection may become much more difficult when you reach the **umbilical cicatrix**. The cicatrix is a tough, short cord structure that connects from the inner surface of skin of the depth of the belly button down to the fascia, giving it the 'inny' appearance. You just need to **divide this** with your scissors if it's in your way and then you can carry on the dissection. Once the whole sac has been dissected out, and the fascia is visible all around the neck, you can decide if you need to **open the sac** (if you haven't already accidentally). You must open it and inspect the contents if you had clinical concern, if say the patient had a tender hernia and was vomiting. If this is just a standard elective day case, you don't need to unless you have trouble reducing the hernia at this stage. Assuming you haven't opened the sac—**poke it back** through the defect in the fascia. If you have opened it, and all is viable, reduce the contents, **close the sac** with absorbable suture such as 2–0 Vicryl and poke that back in. If there is non-viable bowel this will need **resecting** and an end-to-end small bowel anastomosis formed. You may need to **enlarge the defect** either up and down or side to side to get proper access to do this. Usually, however, it's just **omentum** and you may need to divide adhesions that develop between the omentum and the inside of the sac. The last thing you need to do

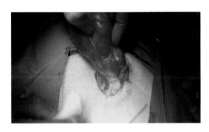

The whole sac has been dissected out and the junction with anterior rectus sheath can be seen.

before repairing the defect is **create a plane** between the **under-surface of the fascia** and the **peritoneum** using scissors extending about 1 cm from the fascial edge all the way around, thus making a little **extraperitoneal pocket**.

So now you need to **fix the defect**. There are two options—**suture** or **mesh**, or both. If large or recurrent: mesh. If small: sutures. There are two options to suturing, firstly you can just do some standard **interrupted sutures** with non-absorbable 1 Nylon for instance or you can do a **Mayo repair** which is much more fun, and has the purported benefit of being a stronger repair. The aim is to make the top fascial edge overlap with the bottom one, also called a **'vest-over-pants'** repair. If the tissues are under too much tension, however, this may not be possible and in fact may be counter-productive. This is how you do it:

1 **Pick up the lateral edges** of your defect with Babcock forceps and get your assistant to elevate them, pulling them laterally, thus making the defect more like a **horizontal slit**.

2 Go through the **superior fascial edge** about 1 cm away from the edge from **outside to inside**.

3 Go through the **inferior fascial edge** about 1 cm away from the edge from **outside to inside**.

4 Go back through the **inferior fascial edge** from **inside to outside** 1 cm along parallel with the fascial edge.

5 Go back through the **superior fascial edge** from **inside to outside** 1 cm along parallel with the fascial edge.

6 Leave the ends **long** and **clip them**.

7 Repeat as many times as needed until the defect length is covered.

8 Pull on all the clips.

9 Gasp in **awe** as the top edge overlaps the bottom one, as though a vest was being pulled over a pair of pants.

Alternatively, you can repair the defect with a **mesh**. The helpful thing about this kind of hernia is that once you've dissected into that space between fascia and peritoneum, you've created a little subfascial pocket to put the mesh

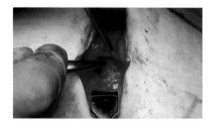

The defect is seen with mesh inserted into the extraperitoneal space.

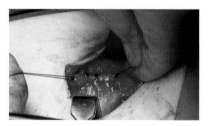

Several interrupted stitches have closed the defect over the mesh.

(a)

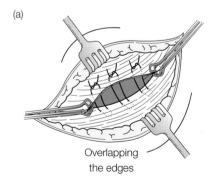

Overlapping the edges

(b)

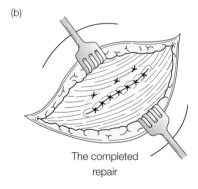

The completed repair

Mayo's operation for the repair of an umbilical hernia.

in, so **shape** and **size** the mesh to **fit** into your **subfascial extraperitoneal pocket**. You can then loosely **close the defect** with 1 Nylon interrupted sutures for instance. Once the patient wakes up and starts going about her usual activities, the abdominal contents **pushes the mesh into apposition** against the fascia. This is called a **sublay mesh**. There's nowhere for that mesh to escape to! It doesn't even need suturing in usually because it can't get out beyond the confines of your pocket! Marvellous!

Of course, if the defect is large and you can't get the fascial edges together without undue tension, the mesh will need to be **sutured to the fascial edges** and the fascial edges not stitched directly together—this is unusual however in paraumbilical hernias—usually the defect is only about 1 cm or so in size. That's something that's needed usually with **large incisional hernias**.

So with the defect closed, all that remains is to **reconstruct the umbilicus** and close. Stitch the base of the cicatrix down onto the fascia from whence it came with a couple of interrupted absorbable sutures. If there's enough superficial fascia/fat to stitch a deep layer so be it, otherwise just **close the skin** with a subcuticular continuous absorbable suture.

Notes

Some people always make their transverse incision well **inferior to the hernia** or the crescentic skin fold. This is also a nice way of doing it; the idea is that you cut down through skin safely, some distance from the sac, aiming straight down to fascia, towards the base of the cicatrix (paraumbilical hernias usually come out above the cicatrix). Once the cicatrix is found they divide it immediately, seeing the sac beyond this; they then proceed in exactly the same way. It has the advantage of a lower and therefore more cosmetic scar.

Rarely, if you're convinced there is dead small bowel in the hernia you might be tempted to do a **vertical incision** over the hernia that you could extend so as to be able to open the abdomen formally as in a laparotomy. Remember, however, if you can do an abdominal aortic aneurysm repair through a transverse incision, you should be fine with a small bowel resection.

Occasionally, the skin overlying the hernia is so thin it looks like purple parchment paper after it's been dissected off. **Resect this skin**, it will only **necrose**, the wound will **break down**, the mesh will get **infected** and **no one will thank you**. In hernias that you pick up preoperatively like these, particularly the very large recurrent ones, discuss with the patient preoperatively that reconstructing the umbilicus may be impossible and get consent that they're happy with that.

Summary

- The extent of the hernia is **marked** pre-operatively with permanent marker
- The patient is under **general anaesthetic** or **spinal** and the abdomen is **shaved**, **prepped** and **draped**
- Make a **curved incision** over the hernia
- **Dissect out the sac** using traction on the superior skin edge and pushing down on the hernia
- **Dissect** down to the **neck**
- **Repeat** on the **inferior edge**, dividing the cicatrix
- Open or don't **open the sac**
- Decide on **viability** of the contents and proceed as appropriate
- **Reduce** the sac
- Make a **subfascial, extraperitoneal pocket**
- **Close the defect** with either sutures or mesh
- **Reconstruct the umbilical pit** by stitching the cicatrix to fascia
- **Close** the skin

7 Appendicectomy

Matt Stephenson and George H C Evans

> **Video** | **14 min 34 s**
> Matt Stephenson, Surgical Registrar*
> Royal Sussex County Hospital, Brighton

Introduction

Older surgeons often like to wax lyrical about how they were sent off to do an appendicectomy on their first day of being a houseman without any supervision or prior training. They apparently did about 1400 appendicectomies in their first year and by the end of 2 months they could finish one in 5 minutes and still have time to have a drag on their pipe, check the cricket score and arrange a date with the scrub nurse. Either rose tinted be their spectacles or they really were a breed apart back then. It's true to say that an appendicectomy can be very straight forward, but if you believe they're all like that, you probably haven't done enough or you're just using a giant wound every time.

Procedure

With the patient **supine** and under **general anaesthetic**, shave and prep the whole of the abdomen but **drape** just the right lower quadrant. Identify **Mc Burney's point**, which is two-thirds of the way from the **umbilicus** to the **anterior superior iliac spine (ASIS)**. A **gridiron** incision is an incision centred on this point but running perpendicular to this line—this is rarely needed and is mainly of historical interest, back in the days when cosmesis was lower on the surgeon's agenda.

Instead, perform a **Lanz** incision, which is centred on the same point but in the line of the skin creases, so essentially

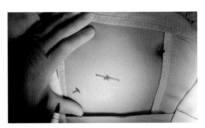

The landmarks of the ASIS and the umbilicus allow you to identify McBurney's point.

---

*A second appendicectomy is shown in the video and this was performed by Rohan Kumar and Christie Swaminatham.

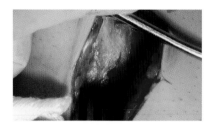

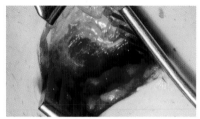

External oblique aponeurosis is exposed in the base of the wound.

The next layer is the internal oblique with its fibres running at 90 degrees to external oblique.

horizontal. A **modified Lanz** is another option, which is the same incision, just slightly lower, for the cosmetic benefit.

Cut through **skin**, **superficial fascia** comprising the fatty-laden **Camper's fascia** and then the more clearly seen thin, whitish layer of **Scarpa's fascia**. Then through **true fat** and look out for the fibres of the **external oblique**, which are coursing inferomedially. Here, insert a self-retaining retractor—such as a **Travers** retractor. Get **haemostasis** as you go with the diathermy.

Make a **small stab incision** in the external oblique and slide your dissecting scissors beneath that layer in both directions creating a space. Then cut the aponeurosis of external oblique with the scissors in both directions in the line of its fibres and insert your retractor into this space.

Next you have to open the **internal oblique** layer—there's a very thin layer of connective tissue around this which is usually easier to just incise, but then you need to split this muscle—here it runs perpendicular to the external oblique. You can open up a space initially with a clip but

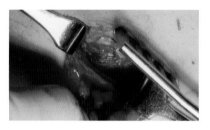

Here in the next layer the fibres are running transversely.

then it's easiest to use Langenbeck retractors. So this is a **muscle splitting** technique. The same needs to be done for the next layer, the **transversus abdominus**, which runs transversely. If the patient is obese there's often a layer of fat in between each of these layers.

After you've opened transversus abdominus you'll come to the **peritoneum** itself, which may be covered by an **extraperitoneal fat** layer. Here you can see the peritoneum as a whitish, often described as glistening, membrane. Put **two clips** on it and **feel** between finger and thumb to check you haven't caught any bowel. Then **snip** the peritoneum with your scissors and allow air to enter the

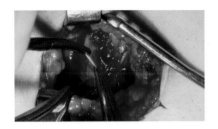

The shiny white peritoneum has been picked up in clips.

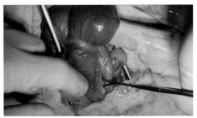

The caecum has been delivered and the appendix is becoming visible—Babcock forceps are now encircling it.

peritoneal cavity—the bowel will then fall away to safety. Note any free fluid and, if there is any, take a **microbiology swab**; also note any free air which you will see as a bubble under the peritoneum. Now **enlarge the whole** in the peritoneum with the scissors and then stretch it with your fingers.

So now we have to find the appendix, which is sometimes easier said than done. First of all, remove your retractor and clips as these just get in the way and put your finger into the peritoneal cavity. **Feel for the appendix**—a tubular structure, maybe there's a mass due to an inflamed appendix and adherent omentum. But the likelihood is you won't feel anything useful at all, at least until you're a bit more experienced at it.

So you need to deliver the appendix into the wound. **Non-traumatic forceps** like **Dennis-Brown forceps** are very useful for this—others prefer using their fingers or **Babcock forceps**. Try to look for the caecum and deliver that out. When reaching in and delivering blindly, which to a certain extent you sometimes have to do, what you will deliver will be one of

three things and none of them are the appendix: **omentum, small bowel** or **caecum**. It's the caecum you want. If you keep getting omentum or small bowel, push it medially out of the way with a swab on a stick. If you're really struggling with small bowel it sometimes helps to ask the anaesthetist to tilt the table to the left so gravity helps tilt the small bowel away. You will recognise the colon by its pale pink colour and presence of those longitudinal **taenia coli**. Once you've got it, trace the taenia coli inferiorly—they converge on the appendix. **Deliver** it into the wound using **Babcock forceps** around the proximal appendix, and another around the distal appendix to secure it.

First you need to **ligate and divide the mesoappendix**. Do this with clipping, cutting and tying, with absorbable ties like 2–0 Vicryl. Now crush the appendix base gently with a clip and then immediately replace the clip just distally to this. **Transfix or tie** the base of the appendix and cut the appendix off flush with the clip, leaving a short stump of appendix. Some people bury the stump with a

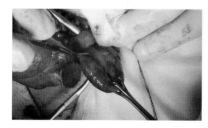

The inflamed appendix is controlled with two Babcock forceps to display the mesoappendix.

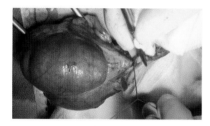

With the mesoappendix completely divided the appendix has been clipped and the base is tied and will then be divided.

purse string suture. Others diathermy the mucosa on the appendix stump. Others do neither of these and leave it as is. There is no strong evidence for any particular choice.

If the appendix was normal, **examine the rest** of the ascending colon, the distal small bowel for a Meckel's diverticulum, the reproductive organs in the woman and anything else you can reach through your small incision. If the appendix was really inflamed with contamination in the abdominal cavity, **wash** the peritoneal cavity out with normal saline. **Close the wound in layers** with absorbable sutures. You may find it helpful to

close the peritoneal layer just because it keeps the bowel from interfering with the rest of the closure but it's not imperative. Close the transversus and internal oblique together with a couple of interrupted stitches just to show them the way and then the external oblique with another continuous stitch. If you have any thread left you may try to close the fat and fascia layer, altogether but this isn't essential. If the appendix was normal or only mildly inflamed close the skin with an absorbable **subcuticular continuous** suture. If it was gangrenous and there was lots of free pus use **skin staples**, the rationale being that it's easier to remove one or two staples in the event of a wound infection than it is to open a wound that's been closed subcuticularly. But not everyone agrees and will always close using subcuticular stitches. Consider giving some **local anaesthetic** depending on whether the anaesthetist's already given a block. Apply a dry dressing like Mepore or Opsite.

Notes

So what do you do if you can't bring out the appendix just like that? Welcome to the club. Well, first of all, the appendix may be **stuck** to some omentum and you will need to feel with your fingers to free it up, particularly if it's a pelvic appendix stuck, say, to the pelvic side wall. You need a little experience to know how much force you can use when blindly trying to free up adhesions, but most adhesions will come away with fairly gentle probing fingers, making it much easier to try again and deliver the appendix.

You'll regret thinking appendicectomies are easy when faced with a 35-stone patient with a high retrocaecal appendix. Firstly, the obese patient will obviously mean that before you've even got to the external oblique, you're already looking down a very deep hole. Try using a **Norfolk and Norwich** self-retainer—like the Travers but with deeper scope. Secondly, always warn patients about this beforehand—you'll almost certainly need a longer incision. Thirdly, there will probably be additional layers of fat in between all the muscle layers and in the preperitoneal space, just anticipate this and make your way through it. Fourthly, even if the caecum and appendix are nicely mobile and easy to deliver out of the wound—in an obese patient that still only means at the bottom of a deep dark hole. You need **good retraction** from your assistant and a **generous sized hole**.

More problematic is the **retrocaecal appendix**. In your exam you will probably get away with saying **'mobilise the caecum'** which means dividing the peritoneum holding down the caecum. You'll need a bigger hole for that so extend the wound. Alternatively, if you can get the base of the appendix but the tip seems to be vanishing off into the distance and you can't deliver it, consider starting by amputating it at the base before you divide the mesoappendix. You then divide the mesoappendix in a retrograde direction. This can make the appendix much

easier to deliver. Bear in mind, however, that the appendix or even just the tip of the appendix can be very friable—you need to take care not to leave chunks of it behind.

Even more problematic is the **subhepatic appendix**. In other words, you've hunted everywhere for it and eventually find that it's coursing up behind the ascending colon and its tip is nestled somewhere in the region of the hepatic flexure. Bummer. Again, there's no two ways about it—you need excellent assistance and a generous sized wound. Many people advocate extending the wound laterally by curving the incision superiorly, creating what looks like a **hockey stick**, or even turning it into something heading towards being a **Rutherford–Morrison** incision, which is a continuation of the lateral end of the wound obliquely up towards the loin. You obviously can't keep to the gentler muscle separation technique you usually use for an appendicectomy—you'll need to just cut through the muscles en masse. With the right exposure, the rest of the operation becomes much easier whatever the position of the appendix.

Remember, if you're struggling, the likeliest problem is that you have inadequate access—make the hole bigger—much better a safe operation at the cost of a larger scar. In fact if you call your boss, the first thing he'll do is extend the wound—you can always do the operation if the hole is big enough. **Remember, big mistakes through small holes**.

Summary

- The patient is **supine** under **general anaesthetic** with the abdomen **shaved** and **prepped** and the right lower quadrant **draped**
- Make a **Lanz** incision over McBurney's point
- **Cut** through **skin, superficial fascia, fat** and identify **external oblique**
- Incise **external oblique** and open with scissors
- Insert a **self-retaining retractor**
- Open **internal oblique** and **transversus abdominus** by a **muscle splitting** technique
- Put clips on the **peritoneum** and **open** this with scissors
- Take a **swab** for microscopy, culture and sensitivity if there's pus
- **Examine** with a **finger**
- Try to **deliver the appendix** into the wound
- Once identified, use **two Babcock forceps** to hold on to the appendix
- **Ligate** and **divide** the **mesoappendix**
- **Transfix** or **tie the stump** and amputate the appendix and send to histology
- **Examine** the small bowel, caecum, pelvic viscera and anything else you can lay your fingers on
- Consider a **washout**
- **Close in layers** with absorbable suture
- **Close the skin** either with **subcuticular** absorbable suture or **skin clips** if heavily infected
- Consider **local anaesthetic** infiltration
- **Remember if you're struggling— you probably need a bigger wound**

8 Establishing a Pneumoperitoneum

Matt Stephenson and Philip Ridings

> **Video** | **5 min 34 s**
> Philip Ridings, Consultant Surgeon
> Royal Sussex County Hospital, Brighton

Introduction

Transverse. Vertical. Curved. Supraumbilical. Infraumbilical. Through the cicatrix. Take your pick. Every boss you work for will do it a different way and insist that theirs is the best. Certainly, like anything, if that's the way you always do it you're bound to look slick. The most important thing is that it's done safely—ensuring that underlying bowel, or worse, aorta, is not injured.

Gynaecologists still tend to prefer the **Verre's** needle technique where a tiny nick is made in the skin and the needle is advanced through the abdominal wall blindly until you feel the 'give' of overcoming the resistance of the peritoneum, then you insufflate blindly into what you hope is the peritoneal cavity. You can then insert your port blindly into what you hope is the insufflated peritoneal cavity. Most general surgeons favour the open **Hasson** technique, whereby you open the layers of the abdominal wall under **direct vision** and actually see the peritoneum and open it. It is precisely how you perform your variation of the Hasson technique which is open for debate. But as long as it is **safe**, reasonably **quick**, **cosmetically acceptable** and is closed properly afterwards to prevent **port site herniation**, it's OK.

Here we'll describe the method shown in the video—a transverse, subumbilical approach.

Procedure

The patient is **supine** (or may be in the **Lloyd–Davies** position if access to the anus or vagina is needed, for instance if you're going to anastomose to the rectum or manipulate the uterus) and under **general anaesthetic**. **Prep** and **drape** the abdomen appropriately to the

How to Operate: for MRCS Candidates and Surgical Trainees, First Edition. M. Stephenson. © 2011 John Wiley & Sons, Ltd.
Published 2011 by John Wiley & Sons, Ltd.

procedure you're planning to perform. Get the **CO₂ tubing**, **diathermy** lead, **camera** lead and **suction** tubing all ready.

Make a **transverse incision** immediately **below the umbilicus** about 1.5 cm long using a fairly pointed blade, either an 11 or 15. Only cut through **skin** and the most **superficial layer** of subcutaneous fat. Bear in mind your anatomy—major structures are not far behind skin in the slim patient. It is not unheard of in the very thin patient, for the unwary, and even the not so unwary, to have inadvertently gone straight through into the aorta. Common sense and care should prevent such a catastrophe. Much of the **dissection** is done **blunt**. So once the incision is made, use **Langenbeck retractors** to open up the tissues overlying the linea alba. In the midline the tissues separate apart very easily. Sometimes you may need to use scissors to help. If the abdominal wall is very thin you may come straight down on to the **linea alba**—a white fibrous layer. Most of the time, however, with the average portly lady requiring her gall-bladder out, this is quite some way away. Therefore, bring the linea alba up to meet you. Insert a heavy clip like a **Kocher** blindly into the wound and grab the first firm tissue it encounters and pull it up. The first few times you try this, you'll probably just pick up bits of fat that fragment, but with a bit of practise you'll be able to tell the difference between this and linea alba. **Pull the linea alba up** close to the surface of the wound and **insert another**

Kocher under direct vision onto the linea alba next to the other one. Position them so they are **either side of the midline**. Use scissors or an 11 blade to make a **vertical hole** in the linea alba, just below the umbilical cicatrix. The peritoneum is immediately below the linea alba at this point with no or minimal preperitoneal fat—so with scissors, **cut this also**. You'll then see the black hole in the peritoneum appear and you can **insert your finger** and **sweep around** to check there are no adhesions and that you've entered the peritoneal cavity.

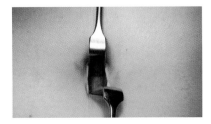

Langenbeck retractors have dissected through the tissues to reveal the white linea alba in the base of the wound.

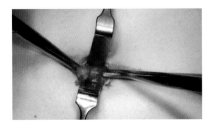

Kochers are lifting up the linea alba either side of the midline.

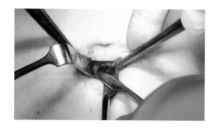

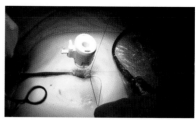

The scissors have made a hole in the peritoneum and by opening the blades the hole is enlarged.

The port has been inserted, the introducer removed and the box stitch tied around it to secure it with one throw.

You could proceed to putting the port straight in, but it's generally easier whilst you have control of the linea alba with your clips to **put in the stitch** to the linea alba that you'll eventually use to close the defect. A **box stitch**, similar to a purse string, is a useful way of doing this, taking two bites of the linea alba on each side of the defect. You can then **insert the port** and pull the suture **fairly tight**, thus closing the tissues around it helping to make an airtight seal. Put **one throw** on the suture and hold it close to the port with a clip.

Regarding the port itself, they vary of course depending on the manufacturer. But in general the consistent elements are that they have an **introducer component** that slips in and out of the port itself. The introducer can be set to two settings—one **'primed'** with a blade and the other **blunt**, where the blade is withdrawn. When the port advances cutting through the tissues the blade cleverly clicks back in when it passes through the abdominal wall thus disarming itself as

soon as it enters the peritoneal cavity, making it blunt. Obviously, you wouldn't therefore want to use a primed port when you've already made a hole, otherwise it will disarm itself on something inside the abdomen you'd rather it didn't. Use the port in the primed setting when you already have the camera in the abdomen and you can see it passing through the abdominal wall safely. Ports also have a side mini port for the **CO_2 tube** to connect to so that the gas can enter the peritoneal cavity. You can turn this mini port on and off in the usual way by twisting the lever.

So once you've introduced your unprimed port into the abdomen, **connect the gas** and turn it on to **low flow**. **Observe** and **percuss** the abdomen to check that it is generally distending and that the gas is getting into the right place, and not for instance into the preperitoneal plane (unless of course you were doing a preperitoneal hernia repair in which case that's the plane you want the gas in, but that's another story). **Insert the camera** for final confirmation that it's the peritoneal cavity and that you're not looking down the lumen of the colon. Switch it onto **high flow** as soon as you're happy it's in the right place. Generally the pressure is kept around 12 mmHg.

Further ports can now be inserted under **direct vision**. Make small **stab incisions**, usually either **5** or **10 mm** depending on the size of the port and insert your primed port through the tissues **watching the tip** of it all the time on the screen.

Then proceed with whatever laparoscopic operation you're doing. But that's enough about that, this isn't a laparoscopic book!

When **closing the port** site, **loosen** the one throw you put on the suture, let all the CO_2 **out** and **withdraw** the ports again under direct vision to check firstly there is **no bleeding** and secondly that **no bowel gets trapped** in them. **Pull** the previously inserted suture **tight** and that should **close the defect** but **check** with a finger. If necessary put another stitch in. Close any other 10 mm port sites in the same way, 5 mm ones don't need to be closed. A **J-shaped needle** mounted at 60 degrees on the needle holder helps to get it down these deep holes. **Close the skin** with an absorbable continuous subcuticular suture.

Summary

- The patient is **supine** or in the **Lloyd–Davies** position under **general anaesthetic**
- **Prep** and **drape**
- Prepare the CO_2, **diathermy**, **camera** and **suction** ready
- Make a **transverse subumbilical** incision
- Open up the tissues with **Langenbeck retractors**
- **Lift up the linea alba** with Kocher retractors
- **Cut the linea alba** and peritoneum between the clips
- Insert a **box stitch** suture
- **Insert non-primed port**
- **Loosely tie** suture around port
- **Connect** CO_2 tubing and turn to **low flow**
- **Confirm position** by observation, percussion and camera inspection
- Turn to **high flow**
- Get on with the operation

9 Laparotomy

Matt Stephenson and Don Manifold

> **Video** | **8 min 20 s**
> Don Manifold, Consultant General and
> Upper GI Surgeon
> Royal Sussex County Hospital, Brighton

Introduction

You may encounter various folk who in an effort to sound clever declare a laparotomy means, specifically, examination of the abdominal contents. You can be pedantic back if you like and explain that *lapar* is the Greek for the fleshy bit between ribs and hips and *otomy* means incising something open. So no, really it's the opening up bit, but in common surgical parlance it tends to mean opening the abdomen and examining what's inside.

Generally, a standard laparotomy is performed these days via a **midline incision**. In the olden days when catgut was all the rage, a laparotomy had to be performed via a paramedian incision. This was because catgut wasn't strong enough to hold the whole abdominal wall together in the midline, each layer had to be closed separately, which had to be off the midline. With the advent of newer suturing techniques paramedian incisions have become more or less obsolete.

For such a simple, common task it's surprising just how quirky different peoples' approaches to opening and closing an abdomen can be. Some people go through each millimetre of tissue meticulously making sure that not one red blood cell escapes, others slice straight down all the way through fascia, open peritoneum in one place and with big scissors chop up and down the wound and then haemostase afterwards. It's largely up to personal preference, style and the indication for the laparotomy. As long as it's done safely, timely and without unnecessary blood loss, it's all good. So with all that said, this is one way to do it.

Procedure

Ensure preinduction **antibiotics** are given if it's expected that contamination may play a role, for instance if bowel is likely to be opened. With the patient **supine** (or **Lloyd–Davies** ('legs up') if you think you may need access to the anus, for instance to insert a circular stapler for rectal

How to Operate: for MRCS Candidates and Surgical Trainees, First Edition. M. Stephenson. © 2011 John Wiley & Sons, Ltd. Published 2011 by John Wiley & Sons, Ltd.

anastomosis) under **general anaesthetic** with a **urinary catheter** *in situ* and the whole of the abdomen **shaved**, **prepped** and **draped**, make a **midline incision** skirting around the umbilicus.

If you predict you're likely to need a left iliac fossa colostomy, skirt to the right. If you predict you're likely to need a right iliac fossa ileostomy, skirt to the left. If you predict neither it doesn't matter. If you're likely to be dealing with upper gastro-intestinal pathology, for example a perforated duodenal ulcer, make the top of the incision higher in the epigastrium. If you're anticipating needing access to the pelvis, for instance in a Hartmann's procedure, make the lower end of the incision close to the pubic symphysis. Anywhere in between, for instance a right hemicolectomy or small bowel pathology, centre the incision at the umbilicus.

Take a scalpel and **incise** the skin in the midline, gently pulling on the abdominal wall towards you with your assistant pulling on the other side with an equal and opposite force. **Tension is key**.

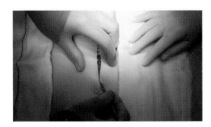

The skin is incised with a knife. The tension on each skin edge can be made with the other hand, or between you and your assistant.

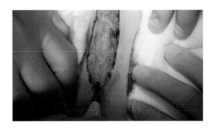

The deep dermis and fat is incised in the midline with diathermy.

Once you're through skin you can swap to **coagulating diathermy** using the blue button on the **monopolar finger switch**—or 'fire stick', or diathermy pencil (or any of its other nicknames). Continue with the diathermy pencil cutting straight down the midline through subcutaneous fat. Provided you stay in the midline this is a relatively **bloodless plane**. For this to be so, it's crucial for you and your assistant to be pulling equally to remain in the middle, an inexperienced assistant may try to pull with the might of an ox to impress you with their keenness.

Eventually, depending on the adiposity of your patient, you will reach the white shiny **linea alba**. Cut straight through this carefully. In very slim patients you will be practically on to the peritoneum after this. More commonly however, the next layer you encounter will be **preperitoneal fat** and this can be quite thick. In just one place of your choosing (around the umbilicus is best), make your way through this, using **blunt dissection**, by opening and closing the jaws of a clip for instance, gradually making a hole in it until you see

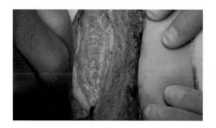

You can see the thick white layer of the linea alba being separated off each side; beneath that is another thick fatty layer, the falciform ligament.

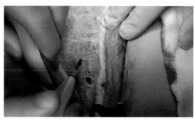

The final layer to be opened is the peritoneum—a small hole can be seen in it already just below and to the right of the diathermy pencil tip.

our old friend **peritoneum**—with its white glistening surface. You may find it helpful to elevate each wound edge with **Lane tissue holding forceps** or just pinching each skin edge with a swab between your fingers.

If after opening the linea alba you encounter vertically running muscle you've drifted off the **linea alba** laterally, one way or the other, through the anterior rectus sheath into the **rectus abdominus**. Don't fear, gently prod around the muscle in the appropriate direction until you find a slim gap between the rectus abdomini. Then proceed as above.

Once you've identified the peritoneum, use **two clips** to pick it up and gently **feel** just below it between finger and thumb to make sure there isn't adherent bowel waiting patiently for an iatrogenic enterotomy (note in the video the patient was slim and the peritoneum very thin—a small hole appeared without any effort thus doing the job for you). **Cut** cautiously between your clips with **scissors** until you've made a hole in it. Poke your

finger in. If pus gushes out to meet you take a **swab** for microscopy, culture and sensitivity (M, C and S). Try not to let it all spill out and contaminate the wound, rather hold up the edges of the peritoneum with your clips and put the sucker in.

With your finger, **sweep** around the inside of the abdominal wall to check for adhesions. In addition to your own finger, get your assistant to help: Tent up the midline with your fingers hooking the abdominal wall up and **diathermy** straight on to the midline tissue (first upwards then downwards, or downwards then upwards, depending on your mood). This way you can safely cut through any remaining fat, rectus sheath or preperitoneal fat and peritoneum safe in the knowledge bowel is out of the way. Be aware of two things. Firstly, as you go further south the rectus abdomini get **very close together** and another oft forgotten muscle—**pyramidalis**—intervenes between them. The plane in the midline can therefore become a little harder to find. Secondly, as you go north you encounter the **falciform ligament** tracing up from the umbilicus to between the right and left lobe of liver. Try to push it to the right of your entry but it doesn't really matter if you cut straight through it.

Generally speaking, the first thing you then need to do after making your hole in the abdominal wall is do a **thorough examination of the abdominal and pelvic contents**. Much of this is done by **touch** alone (and therefore doesn't show up very well on video). You may develop your own system but most people will start by feeling in the right upper quadrant for the liver.

So start by sliding your hand up in to the **right upper quadrant** with the back of your hand pressed against the inside of the abdominal wall (some traditionalists will advocate sliding it in palm up against the abdominal wall and then pronating when over the liver. This has the purported benefit of your fingernails not catching and traumatising the liver edge. Decide for yourself whether you think this makes sense given that as a surgeon you have cut your nails and still have to rotate your hand inside the abdomen directly over the liver).

- Feel the **right lobe** right over its surface up to the diaphragm
- Feel the **falciform ligament** and then the **left lobe** of the liver all over its surface
- Feel the **gallbladder** for stones or rubberiness (inflammation)
- Move your hand up to the back of the left upper quadrant and very gently feel for the **spleen**

- Feel over the anterior surface of the stomach up to the **diaphragmatic hiatus** up in the most superior part of the abdominal cavity where you can feel a short segment of **abdominal oesophagus**
- Feel all parts of the **stomach**—fundus, body, lesser curve, greater curve antrum and pylorus
- Follow the pylorus down to the **duodenum**
- Continue laterally to feel over the retroperitoneal **right kidney** and then feel back over the length of the **pancreas;** to do this it's usually easier to lift the transverse colon and **omentum** superiorly (examining the latter as you do so)
- Continue in the same direction to feel the retroperitoneal **left kidney**
- Now examine the rest of the gut tube starting with the **ligament of Treitz**— where the fourth part of the duodenum is suspended (and serves technically as the division between upper and lower GI bleeding)
- Deliver out all of the bowel and trace it proximally until you find the ligament of Treitz and then trace it all the way down its length from **jejunum** to **ileum** to the **ileocaecal junction**—examine the bowel itself for size, wall thickness and fat encroachment etc., and also the **mesentery** with its **vessels**
- With the mesentery fully delivered, palpate the **aorta** at the root of the mesentery and follow this down to the **iliac arteries**
- Continue along the **colon** noting the **appendix** and follow it up the **ascending**, **transverse** and **descending** colon

down to the rectum feeling it as far down close to the pelvic floor as you can; remember the place where pathology is missed in the colon is the harder to reach splenic flexure (but take great care here—tiny tears of the attachments to the spleen can result in significant haemorrhage and great embarrassment if you have to remove the spleen)

- Whilst in the pelvis, examine the **bladder** and in the very thin, the **ureters**
- Examine the **internal hernial orifices**
- In a woman examine the **uterus**, the **ligaments**, **tubes** and **ovaries**
- If this is an exploratory laparotomy and you've found nothing abnormal—**open the lesser sac** (see *Gastrectomy* chapter) to properly assess the pancreas and check for a posterior perforated gastric ulcer

Now, when have you ever seen anyone doing this thorough a laparotomy? This technique of exploratory laparotomy was entirely the norm in the pre-CT days. Now, most patients go to theatre with a clinical and three-dimensional imaging-driven diagnosis. However, always remember that CTs can be wrong and miss things. Think how many points you'll score over the radiologists if you've identified something they should have spotted. But also remember that patients can have dual pathology. Think how silly you'll look if you patch up your patient's duodenal ulcer only for them to re-present 3 months later with an obstructing rectosigmoid cancer. Also in some exploratory laparotomies you have no idea what's going on, especially in the case of trauma.

Doing a proper exploratory laparotomy takes practise. Why not therefore adopt this as your standard practice? The only caveats to all this is in the presence of obvious malignancy, you don't want to prod an obvious cancer and then rummage all around the abdomen potentially seeding it all over the place. It may sound odd, but if you know there's cancer there, don't touch it until last. Don't overhandle tissues—you could damage them, or in the case of small bowel increase the risk of ileus and potentially adhesions. Also, don't allow localised contamination to become generalised contamination.

Before closing, ensure **haemostasis** and depending on what you've just done, consider **washing out** the peritoneal cavity with some warmed fluid. Warmed normal saline is fine. There is a theoretical argument for using warmed sterile water as this will theoretically cause any tumour cells to swell due to osmotic pressure and lyse. Make sure that the viscera are replaced where they should be and, for instance, the small bowel isn't twisted on its mesentery and the omentum lies over the abdominal contents as before.

The use of **abdominal drains** is highly contentious and different surgeons will vehemently argue for or against them in certain circumstances, so being dogmatic about this is impossible. In general, many surgeons will insert a drain into either an obviously contaminated part of the peritoneal cavity to drain any residual muck, or to an area where they're worried contamination may quickly occur, so it can then be controlled, for instance following insertion of a biliary T-tube where there is concern there may be leakage around the tube.

Closing the abdomen is much easier than it was in the olden days. It's over 30 years now since single-layer continuous **mass closure** was first described and it is now standard practice. Again there are subtle differences in individual technique but here we describe a way that works very well.

Inspect the wound edge and identify the true **fascial layer** of where the rectus sheaths join in the middle—the **linea alba**. This is the important layer to close properly. Peritoneum, fat and muscle are bystanders and get caught up in the process. You may find in the middle that you can see muscle, as on entry you may have skirted slightly off the midline and then have anterior and posterior rectus sheath separated by rectus abdominus. Just make sure you catch both anterior and posterior layers. Take a **1-cm bite** of tissue and keep the stitches **1 cm apart**. **Jenkin's rule** states that the total length

of the suture closing the wound should be at least four times the length of the wound. Most people use a **blunt needle** as this reduces risk to injury of your fingers and to bowel, especially in a tight abdomen, but some prefer sharp.

Most people use a **looped suture**, this makes it easy to thread the needle back through the first loop thus securing it. The slowly absorbable polydioxanone suture (PDS) is a popular choice. Start at either end and work towards the middle. On reaching the middle, tie the two ends together. To make the knot invert and not poke out of the skin of a thin person, make sure the two ends are on the inside of the fascia. Several throws are needed for PDS as it's so slippery.

NB it is not enough to get 24 out of your 25 sutures well placed. If you leave a gap it can become the leading point for a dehiscence or late incisional hernia with all its consequent morbidity—be meticulous.

All that remains is to **close the skin**, which can be done with a subcuticular continuous absorbable suture in most cases, or in the event of significant contamination use clips or even leave the skin open and pack the wound if it was gross faecal contamination (the wound will become infected anyway).

Notes

We've described opening a virgin abdomen. If you're doing a re-do laparotomy (even if four decades ago) you need to take great care to avoid any bowel that's stuck up by adhesions to the posterior

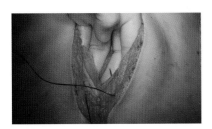

The closure has started from the inferior end of the wound. Take 1-cm bites at 1-cm intervals.

aspect of the abdominal wall (especially in the danger period of roughly 10 days to 2 months after a laparotomy where the adhesions are at their unfriendliest). Also expect the layers to be distorted by previous scar tissue. You may find it easier to enter the peritoneum just above or below the old scar.

If you're having difficulties closing because the bowels keep pushing out, check with the anaesthetist that the muscles are still relaxed. If you're still struggling, consider using a flexible plastic visceral retractor called (and shaped like) a **fish**. It's withdrawn once the closure is almost complete.

Summary

- The patient is positioned **supine** or **'legs up'** under general anaesthetic
- **Shave**, **prep** and **drape** the abdomen
- Make a **midline skin incision** with a **knife**
- Use **diathermy** to divide in the midline through **fat**
- Divide **linea alba** with **diathermy**
- **Pick up peritoneum** and **open**
- **Open rest of wound** protecting bowel
- Perform thorough **exploration**
- **Perform operation**, whatever that may be
- Consider **washout** and **drains** depending on situation
- Ensure **haemostasis** and **return viscera** to their rightful place
- Perform **mass closure**
- **Close skin**

10 Long Saphenous Vein Stripping

Matt Stephenson and Mike Brooks

Video | 9 min 29 s
Mike Brooks, Consultant Vascular Surgeon
Royal Sussex County Hospital, Brighton

Introduction

Once upon a time, varicose vein operations were everywhere on day surgery and in-patient lists. You couldn't move for them. Then many Primary Care Trusts began to 'ration' their services somewhat, moving varicose veins into the low priority group, meaning surgery would only be funded if it were causing significant secondary skin changes. This, combined with the rise of endovenous therapies, means that they have become a relative rarity. Quel dommage! It's a very enjoyable operation, still of course practiced by many in the private sector... What better reasons to get good at it?

There are basically two types of primary operation for varicose veins—one for the long saphenous vein, one for the short (see *Short Saphenous Vein Ligation* Chapter 11). More commonly now, most patients have a duplex scan of the venous system preoperatively to document clearly the pattern of venous incompetence, regardless of whether they have had any of the common risk factors for deep vein thrombosis (DVT) (deep venous obstruction being an absolute contraindication to varicose vein surgery). This makes good sense given the high variability in venous anatomy and possible litigation in cases of potentially avoidable recurrence. Bosses differ *ad nauseum* on their views of selective versus universal preoperative duplex. But considering we operate now on far fewer varicose veins, it would hardly seem that burdensome on your vascular laboratory service to make such requests for the few patients eligible for funding.

Procedure

Preoperatively it is crucial to **mark the veins accurately**. Ask the patient to **stand** up and in good lighting draw lines with permanent marker pen on all the varicose veins. **Be meticulously**

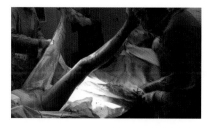

This lady has bilateral long saphenous varicose veins. The whole of the legs are prepped.

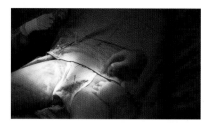

In this case both groins are exposed for bilateral stripping. Palpating the femoral artery pulsation helps guide where to make your incision.

accurate. Ask the patient if there are any you've missed out that are particularly bothering them. If you don't mark them accurately, you will truly hate yourself during the procedure when you fail to find any veins. With the patient in the **Trendelenburg position** (legs up to empty the veins) under **general anaesthetic**, **prep** from the groin down to the ankle, front and back. Wrap the foot in a drape and **drape** from above the groin.

Make a **transverse incision** in the groin crease starting over the medial edge of the femoral pulse and going medially. It only needs to be an inch or so.

Deepen the incision through **superficial fascia** and **fat**. Insert a **Travers** retractor and lift vertically—this will aid your dissection. Using scissors and non-toothed DeBakey forceps gradually **dissect down** looking for a **big fat vein** running vertically in your wound. Once you've found it, it's likely to be the long saphenous vein—can't promise it though—it may not even be big or fat when it's empty bear in mind. You'll need to do some digging around to confirm it. Gradually **dissect** around the vein, keeping close to it. Any veins going transversely, joining it or otherwise can be **ligated** and **divided**. Your aim is to find the **saphenofemoral junction**. The long saphenous vein goes up the leg and then turns deeply in an almost 90 degree bend to join the femoral vein. There is therefore, always a very obvious junction. You need to see this junction to know that you are definitely ligating the long saphenous and not the femoral vein. You may scoff and retort 'nonsense, of course this is the long saphenous vein', but stripping the femoral vein by accident has been done.

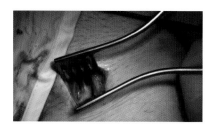

The long saphenous vein has been exposed; note the tributaries.

Ligate and **divide** all the tributaries to the long saphenous vein with absorbable suture such as 2–0 Vicryl. Once you are clearly standing in front of a carefully dissected out saphenofemoral junction with all tributaries divided, it's safe to ligate and divide the long saphenous vein, flush with the femoral vein with a strong absorbable ligature such as 0 Vicryl. Make a small hole in the long saphenous vein, or open the cut end of the vein with two mosquito forceps and **pass the stripper** down it. The stripper is simply a long metallic or plastic wire with a small rounded tip on either end. The strippers come with a selection of different size caps that can be attached to the top end of the wire to assist in avulsing the vein from its bed. However, most surgeons don't use these anymore as they did cause more collateral damage and required a large incision at the bottom end

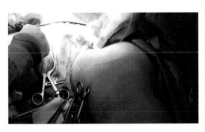

The stripper has been introduced into the top of the left long saphenous vein.

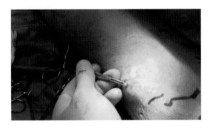

A small incision has been made over the palpable tip of the stripper which is then coaxed out with a clip.

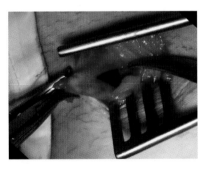

All the tributaries have been divided (note the clips remain on the long saphenous vein side of the ligation thus saving time tying fewer knots. The long saphenous vein has been gently tented up to inspect its junction with the femoral vein (which unfortunately you can't see in this picture).

to extract the vein. Pass the stripper down to **just below the knee**. You can see it and feel it under the skin making its merry way. Sometimes it goes the wrong way down a less significant tributary or gets stuck at a junction, so it may need a little encouragement. Don't force it though. When you can see it/feel it just below the knee, make a small (3–5mm) incision over it. Use a **clip** and **grab hold** of the tip of the stripper and coax this out. Make a small incision in the vein to allow the tip of the stripper out and pull it through a few centimetres. Now tie the top of the vein very firmly around the stripper in the groin with a strong absorbable suture.

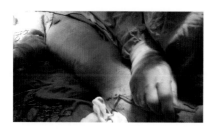

The long saphenous vein has been stripped out from below and has been inverted in the process.

Now to **strip the vein**. Pull on the lower end of the stripper so that the small cap on the top of the stripper engages around the top of the vein. **Pull**. Watch with pleasure as the long saphenous vein pulls out through your inferior hole, usually inverting in the process. Some people do this the other way round, putting the cap on the inferior end and pulling from above. Whatever. You may worry about all the other little tributaries entering into the long saphenous vein in the thigh that you've neither seen or ligated. Don't fear, they may bleed but will give up after a while, firm pressure with a swab over the medial thigh will help reduce the postoperative bruising from this.

So, the long saphenous vein is ligated and stripped—hurrah! That's half the battle won, but what of all these other marks you've made where there were varicose veins that weren't even along the course of the long saphenous vein. These tributaries to the long saphenous vein require **multiple stab avulsions** (MSAs). Take a very thin blade, a Beaver blade (used for corneal surgery) is ideal or otherwise an 11 blade and make a **tiny vertical stab** incision (<2 mm) just next to the mark you made preoperatively. Using a **vein hook**, try to **hook out the vein**, much like trying to dig out a worm from your garden. In fact nothing like that, but the veins are a bit like worms. Once you see a worm appearing in your hook, grasp it with a small clip like a mosquito. Gently try to tease it up. Obviously there are two ends to the worm you're pulling out, usually one going up and one going down. Try to grab each end individually and gently pull it out, keeping on replacing a clip close to the skin so as to reduce the chance of tearing it. **It will tear** eventually though of course; you can't strip long lengths of vein like this but you can then do another stab incision a little way down the marked vein from the last one and repeat. This way, long lengths of vein can be avulsed through multiple tiny (can't really even be seen as scars with time) stabs. Even if you don't get a continuous length of vein, you're **disrupting** it, which does the job. Again, if you pull out a segment of a vein blindly in this way, you are leaving two ends to bleed. They will

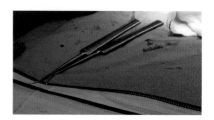

Vein hooks, they come in different sizes.

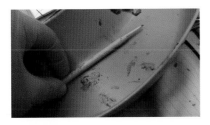

A Beaver blade.

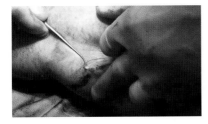

The vein being hooked out.

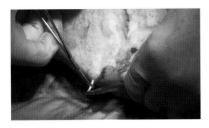

Once the vein can be seen, get a clip on it firmly.

stop, but **pressure** here with a swab will help.

Close the groin wound with absorbable suture to close the **cribriform fascia** (which the long saphenous vein was passing through—closing this layer should at least theoretically reduce the chance of the femoral vein remarrying to another superficial vein). And then the same for the fat/superficial fascia if there's much of it and **subcuticular** absorbable suture to skin. The multiple stab avulsion wounds need only a **steristrip**. Put a **dressing** on the groin wound. **Wrap the leg** firmly with gauze and crepe or similar. This should stay on until the next day, after which the patient can change to wearing stockings day and night for 1 week. Then the dressings can come off and they can switch to wearing stockings only during the day for the following 3 weeks. Encourage them to do plenty of walking, starting the next day.

Notes

If you can't hook out a vein during your MSAs, either you've marked them inaccurately and there isn't a vein there, or you need to improve your hooking skills, which only comes with practise; eventually you'll reach a Zen like state where you sense exactly where the veins are under the skin. Often you can hook the vein out but it crumbles with the slightest traction. These **friable veins** are common and a nuisance, especially with recurrent varicose veins or if the patient has had phlebitis in the past. Persevere, you may need more stabs. At least if the vein is disrupted it may be sufficient to destroy the varicosity locally. Sometimes, especially with thin patients, many veins are visible through the skin whilst on the operating table. Don't be tempted to get all of them, just concentrate on the ones you've marked—the patient just has translucent skin—leave them with some veins.

Summary

- **Mark** the veins very carefully
- Make a **skin crease incision** in the groin
- **Deepen** to find the **long saphenous vein**
- **Dissect** out the long saphenous vein
- Identify the **saphenofemoral junction**
- **Ligate** all tributaries
- **Ligate** the long saphenous vein flush with the femoral vein and **divide**
- Pass the **stripper**
- Make a **small incision** over the tip of the stripper
- **Extract the tip** of the stripper with a clip
- **Tie the top end of the vein firmly to the stripper**
- Pull on the lower end of the stripper, thus **stripping the vein**
- **Press** with a swab over the medial thigh
- Make a **tiny stab** over a marked vein
- **Hook vein out** with a vein hook
- Use a **clip** to pull each end out
- **Repeat** as many times as necessary
- **Close the groin**—absorbable suture to cribriform fascia and fat, then to skin; dry dressing
- **Steristrips** to MSAs
- **Gauze ± wool and crepe** to entire leg

11 Short Saphenous Vein Ligation

Matt Stephenson and Mike Brooks

> **Video** | **5 min 26 s**
> Mike Brooks, Consultant Vascular Surgeon
> Royal Sussex County Hospital, Brighton

Introduction

For a discussion about varicose vein surgery in general see *Long Saphenous Vein Surgery* Chapter 10.

Dealing with the short saphenous vein (SSV) is rather different from the long. The first difference being that most people **don't strip** the short saphenous vein, they just ligate it at its junction with the popliteal vein and may just remove a small segment of it. The main reason for this is that it still works well, and that the sural nerve runs close by, which if you injure it may give the patient a numb calf and lateral part of the foot, and leave you with an awkward phone call to your medical defence society.

Because the level of the saphenopopliteal junction is variable, it is mandatory to do a **preoperative Doppler (a duplex may be preferable if the junction is complex) to confirm the exact location**, otherwise it can be like searching for a needle in a haystack. If the junction's been marked properly, the operation should be straightforward. All the other varicose veins must also be marked as these will have to be dealt with by multiple stab avulsions.

Procedure

The patient is **prone, with head-down tilt on the table** and under **general anaesthetic**. The **saphenopopliteal junction has been marked**. **Prep** and **drape** the popliteal fossa, centred on your mark.

Make a **transverse skin incision** over the mark. Deepen the wound to the popliteal fascia—the deep fascial layer—and hold the skin edges apart with a self-retaining retractor, such as a Travers retractor. Incise the **popliteal fascia** vertically, that is perpendicular to the skin incision and hold the edges apart with clips—you've now entered the popliteal fossa.

How to Operate: for MRCS Candidates and Surgical Trainees, First Edition. M. Stephenson. © 2011 John Wiley & Sons, Ltd. Published 2011 by John Wiley & Sons, Ltd.

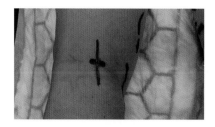

The cross marks the transverse and vertical levels of the saphenopopliteal junction.

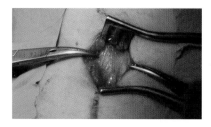

The popliteal fascia has been opened and held apart with clips—the popliteal fossa lies beneath.

Dissect gently through the **popliteal fossa** to find a vertically running vein and follow this up and down using scissors and forceps. Provided you've made your incision roughly where the mark was, that vein is likely to be the **short saphenous vein**. Follow it up and it will gradually be moving deeper and deeper. There maybe a proximal extension of the SSV, called the Giacomini vein, but your preoperative duplex scan should have forewarned you of this. It really helps to have a very thorough scan beforehand and have the result available to you in theatre as the anatomy is variable (much more so

than the saphenofemoral junction in the groin) and there are some nasty bits of anatomy around—and nothing comes with a label on it! The SSV usually passes between the tibial and common peroneal nerves, which must be retracted very carefully to each side, before eventually meeting with another chunkier, deeper vein, also running vertically. You've probably found the **saphenopopliteal junction**. Dissect around it to **confirm the anatomy** and look for any side branches. The gastrocnemius vein(s) often enter the SSV just proximal to the short saphenopopliteal junction

Take right-angled forceps like **Lahey** forceps and get these around the short saphenous vein: **ligate and divide it**. Hold up the ligated end of short saphenous vein that's in continuity with the junction and dissect around it until you're clearly around the junction (without tenting up the popliteal vein too much)—ligate and divide it here, **flush with the junction**, thus excising a short segment of vein.

Close up the **popliteal fascia** if it's not too thin and friable—otherwise an

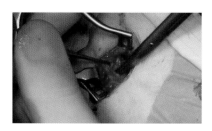

The short saphenous vein has been dissected out and is held in forceps, and is about to be ligated.

unsightly bulge develops. Ensure **haemostasis** and **close the fat** and then the **skin** with continuous absorbable sutures.

If the patient needs any **avulsions** of other veins, proceed as in *Long Saphenous Vein Surgery* Chapter 10.

Summary

- Ensure accurate **preoperative marking** of the saphenopopliteal junction and varicose veins
- The patient is **prone, head down and** under **general anaesthetic**
- **Prep** and **drape**
- Incise the **skin transversely** over the mark
- Incise the **popliteal fascia vertically**
- **Dissect** out the **short saphenous vein**
- **Avoid damaging the nerves**
- Identify the **saphenopopliteal junction**
- **Confirm the anatomy**
- **Ligate and divide** the short saphenous vein
- Ligate and divide the short saphenous vein **at the short saphenopopliteal junction**
- Ensure **haemostasis**
- **Close** the **popliteal fascia**
- **Close** the **fat** and **skin**
- Perform **avulsions** if needed

12 Abdominal Aortic Aneurysm Repair

Matt Stephenson and Mike Brooks

> **Video** | **15 min 4 s**
> Mike Brooks, Consultant Vascular Surgeon
> Royal Sussex County Hospital, Brighton

Introduction

One of the big three index vascular operations, the aortic aneurysm repair, is one of those major operations seen less and less as **endovascular aneurysm repair** (**EVAR**) has increased in popularity. This has meant not only fewer chances to see one, but also they've tended to be the more complex cases, which aren't amenable to EVAR because of their anatomical configuration, for example a short angulated neck where you can't land an endovascular stent or heavily diseased tortuous iliac arteries through which you can't negotiate a stent. Whilst you're not likely to be asked to do a ruptured abdominal aortic aneurysm (AAA) on your own on your first surgical attachment, everyone who might be called to assist with one needs to know the steps—they can get pretty frenetic in the ruptured situation, which is more or less the same procedure as the elective situation except for the higher potential for soiling oneself.

Procedure

The patient is **supine** under **general anaesthetic** with central venous pressure and arterial monitoring. An epidural and a urinary catheter have been sited. The whole of the abdomen is **shaved** and **prepped including the groins** (in case access to the femoral arteries is needed later). Make either a standard **midline laparotomy** (see *Laparotomy* Chapter 9) or a **transverse incision** in the epigastrium; the latter will be explained here. It's not advisable to do a transverse incision if you anticipate (based on the preoperative CT) that you might have to extend the graft into the iliacs as you'll struggle to reach them.

Make an incision through **skin**, **superficial fascia** and **fat** and identify the **anterior rectus sheath**. **Incise the**

How to Operate: for MRCS Candidates and Surgical Trainees, First Edition. M. Stephenson. © 2011 John Wiley & Sons, Ltd.
Published 2011 by John Wiley & Sons, Ltd.

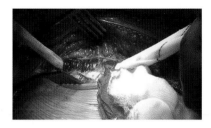

The right rectus abdominus has been elevated with a swab to safely divide it.

anterior rectus sheath and **identify the two rectus abdominus muscles**. Pass a long Robert clip underneath each muscle in turn and use the tassel of a large swab to elevate each muscle away from the posterior rectus sheath. Use monopolar diathermy to **divide each muscle** taking care to buzz or ligate the superior epigastric artery and any of its branches. Then pick up the **posterior rectus sheath** with two clips and **open it** (this usually opens the peritoneum too but this may need to be opened separately). **Extend the wound laterally** in both directions, if necessary, for adequate exposure, beyond the lateral limit of the rectus sheath cutting straight through the lateral abdominal wall muscles. Now perform a **laparotomy** examination as standard.

You now need to **find the aneurysm**. To do this deliver the small bowel out of the abdomen to the patient's right. To prevent heat and fluid loss the bowel can be wrapped in wet swabs and placed in a plastic bag—this will also prevent fluid leaking through to your underwear if you've not taken the precaution of wearing something waterproof. Alternatively, the bowel maybe packed within the abdominal cavity on the right side. **Following the small bowel mesentery to its root** on the left hand side you'll discover a large, pulsating mass in the retroperitoneum, this is the aneurysm sac. So, the sac is covered by **peritoneum** and you need to get through this layer to get on to the aneurysm sac proper. The top of the infrarenal aorta is crossed by another structure—the **duodenum**—and this usually needs to be mobilised first so it can be retracted superiorly and laterally. Great care needs to be taken at this stage as any injury to the duodenum or other bowel could be catastrophic as you potentially will contaminate the new graft and predispose to an aortoenteric fistula. Getting decent exposure of the whole of the aneurysm is crucial and, whilst in the past this has required two exhausted and bored juniors or students, fortunately there is now a very useful self-retaining retractor—the **Omnitract**—which does all the hard work of retraction for you (and

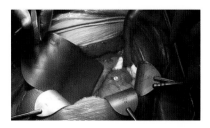

Omnitract has been inserted, retracting small bowel to the right (which has been packed inside) and the colon superiorly and laterally.

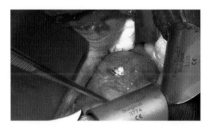

Note the duodenum coursing obliquely over the front of the aneurysm.

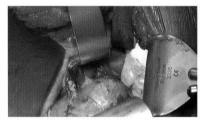

The duodenum has been dissected off the front of the aneurysm to reveal the aneurysm neck.

doesn't complain nor need refreshment). It does need readjusting as you develop your access with the following steps.

So **start at the top**. There is usually* a clear plane between the duodenum and the aneurysm—divide **between the two** using diathermy or sharp dissection **lifting the duodenum superiorly** and **exposing the front of the neck** of the aneurysm. With the duodenum safely out of the way dissect **down onto the neck** of the aneurysm through the periadventitial layers. Ideally, you want to go high enough up to visualise the roots of the renal arteries coming off on each side. The main structure to be mindful of is the **left renal vein**, which crosses transversely at

around this level.** Once identified **retract it superiorly;** rarely, if it's obstructing access it may need to be **ligated** and **divided**. With the front of the neck clear gently **dissect down each side** of the neck, keeping in the plane close to the aneurysm. There will be lots of vascular periadventitial tissue so maintain **meticulous haemostasis** as you go. This stage is done by **diathermy** and **gentle blunt dissection** with, for instance, the tip of the sucker, until the tip of your **finger** can feel the front of the **vertebral body** on each side of the neck. You do *not* need to get round the back of the aneurysm, don't even think about it—essentially just make a space on each side of the neck into which you can get the jaws of your clamp.

With the top of the aneurysm dissected to give enough space to get a clamp on, **dissect inferiorly** over the front of the aneurysm sac through the **peritoneum** and **periadventitial tissues** to keep in the plane just around the sac proper. On reaching the bottom of the aneurysm, dissect left and right to identify the **common iliac arteries**. In the same way as the neck of the aneurysm, dissect **each side of each common iliac artery** to make a plane to accommodate the jaws of the clamp. If these are also aneurysmal, keep dissecting distally until you reach normal-calibre vessel. Again, you do not need to go around the back of the vessels, doing so can be very hazardous— remember that the iliac veins are right behind and injury to these can result in disastrous bleeding.

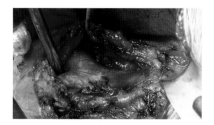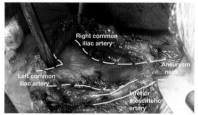

Side-on view of the aneurysm with the retroperitoneum dissected off.

You've now made spaces to get **proximal control** at the neck of the aneurysm and **distal control** around each common iliac. Ask the anaesthetist to kindly administer 3 to 5000 units of heparin intravenously (the exact dose should vary depending on the patient's weight) and wait 3 minutes before applying your clamps (in practice, therefore, you ask for the heparin whilst you're still tidying up your clamp spaces and choosing which clamps you're going to use).

Apply the clamp around the neck of the aneurysm; palpate the sac to check that it's **no longer pulsating**. Apply a clamp around each **common iliac artery**, you now have proximal and distal control and you're ready to open the sac. Your assistant should be ready with **suction** and the scrub nurse should have a **2–0 non-absorbable suture** ready to pass to your hand (you'll see why shortly). Use a knife and **incise the sac** from superior to inferior. Inside the sac you'll probably find a mass of unsightly substance—**old thrombus** (there can be a variable amount which can all be scooped out), there is the **blood** that was sitting in the aneurysm at the time of clamping and—*what's this?*—**blood pouring** into the back of the aneurysm sac. You thought you had control. There's almost always **back bleeding from the lumbar arteries** which run directly off the back of the aorta. Sometimes, also the **inferior mesenteric artery** is still patent. Your assistant speedily **sucks** up the blood and you **rapidly suture** closed the **ostia of these lumbar arteries** (highly variable but on average three to five of them) and also of the **inferior mesenteric artery**, or this can be slinged.***

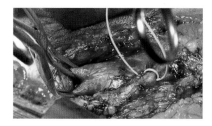

Both iliacs have been clamped and a silastic sling is controlling the inferior mesenteric artery in case it back bleeds.

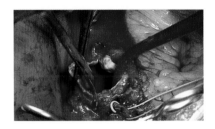

Viewing from below—the sac has been opened. Scissors are dividing up to the neck and down to the iliacs.

The inside of the sac is now dry and you need to **fashion the neck** of the aneurysm to suture your **graft** to. To do this, use scissors to cut up the sac towards the level of normal calibre and then cut laterally in both directions to about **half the circumference** of the neck. **Do the same inferiorly** to either normal calibre aorta or, more likely, the origins of the common iliacs. If the common iliacs are aneurysmal you'll need to follow them down until you reach normal calibre and open the sac to a hemicircumference as with the neck. Now decide which graft to put in and use a **sizer** to check the diameter of the neck. If you're plumbing onto aorta inferiorly, or the origins of the iliacs, use a **straight graft**, if onto the iliacs separately—a **trouser graft**.

Suture the **top end of the graft first**. Many people use a **parachute technique** using a non-absorbable suture such as **double ended 2–0 Prolene**. So, begin by going through the **sac wall from inside to outside** at about **3 o'clock** (if you imagine looking up at the neck from below). Then **go outside to inside** on the graft. **Leave the suture loose** for now. Then go back in through the **inside of the sac wall** and **outside of the graft** in a **clockwise direction** until the back of the anastomosis is completed. Then **parachute** the graft down into position by pulling each end of the thread with equal and opposite tension allowing the graft to bed down. Make sure there are no loose stitches. Carry on with the same suture until you reach the front of the aorta, then use the other end, remembering to pass the needle first through the graft again, always passing inside to outside on the aorta. **Complete the front of the anastomosis**. This is not a delicate anastomosis as with, for example, a radiocephalic fistula. The bites need to take strong tissue (each bite must included the adventitia which is the only layer with any strength—anything less will pull out), and have no big gaps—remember systemic blood pressure's about to pump through this anastomosis. With the anastomosis completed place a new clamp occluding the graft and slowly ease off the proximal clamp *(don't take it right out though!)*. Press a swab gently over the anastomosis as you do so. Provided the wound doesn't now well up with blood (in which case squeeze back on the clamp) remain in this pose until the song finishes on the radio. Then take a look. If it's leaking, even if it looks like a bit of a spurter, reapply your swab around the anastomosis and wait until the end of the next song (perhaps not Bohemian

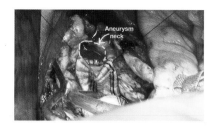

Viewing from below—the back row of sutures of the proximal anastomosis has been put in.

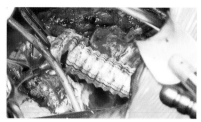

Viewing from the side again—the back row of the distal anastomosis to the iliacs has been completed.

Rhapsody). During this time the **tension in the suture will be equalising** all around the anastomosis closing up loose patches and clot will be forming in other leaky areas. Only if after the second song does it not stop bleeding will you have to think about putting in some **extra stitches**. The commonest problem is a lack of tension in the suture line, sometimes caused by the suture cutting through the thrombus or atheroma in the wall and sometimes due to the incompetence of your sleepy assistant. The simplest solution is to hook the loose suture up using a nerve hook, pass a 2/0 Prolene through this loop and then tie this to a second Prolene suture that you have inserted through the anastomosis and tied at the same point.

Now **measure up the graft** for length so it will fit snugly to where your distal anastomosis will be. Too loose and it will tent up when blood starts pumping through it, too short and you will be cursing the day you chose vascular surgery as a career. Do the **distal anastomosis** in just the same way as the proximal. Just before

you tie the suture, very gently ease off each of the iliac clamps in turn to allow some **back bleeding** and **remove any clot** sitting in the iliac arteries. Also flush downwards by temporarily loosening the clamp on the graft, then **flush** the inside of the graft with **heparinised saline**.

You're now ready to **'leg the legs in'. Warn your anaesthetist**, there may be profound metabolic shifts that may need rapidly dealing with by fluid administration, tinkering with drugs and cursing. There are various ways of letting go with the clamps. One way is to **ease off the left iliac artery** and assess whether just the back bleeding is enough to make your anastomosis leak. Then **ease off on the clamp** which is on your **graft**. Repeat the waiting game you played with the proximal clamp if it's leaking. Finally **let in the right leg** when the anaesthetist is ready. Check the femoral pulses have returned. Alternatively you can release both iliac clamps but keep your fingers clenched around the graft after you've removed the top clamp, then gradually ease off as the blood pressure allows. Although your fingers will give you a good idea about how good, or bad, the systemic pressure is, it's always worth being able to see the invasive systolic blood pressure on the monitor as you do this release, so ask your friendly anaesthetist to angle the screen towards you. You will normally find that he or she has put down the crossword or Sudoku at this point of the operation so you'll have their attention.

Sort out **haemostasis** and then **close the aneurysm sac** and then the peritoneum with some absorbable suture such as 2–0 Vicryl to protect your graft. By this time the **femoral pulses** should be palpable and ask for someone to lift the drapes over the feet and check they look OK before closing. They hopefully will be able to feel pedal pulses (if they were there pre op), or detect them with a Doppler.

Close the abdomen with a **mass closure technique** using a **non-absorbable suture such as Nylon**. Aneurysms are the exception to the usual PDS/Maxon (slowly absorbable) treatment as patients with aneurysms have a higher tendency to get incisional hernias (probably due to the defective collagen that helped give them their aneurysm). Close the skin with **subcuticular absorbable sutures** or clips. Always look at the feet towards the end of the procedure to check these have not become ischaemic from an embolus flying off during the operation. If this has happened they will need an immediate embolectomy via the femoral artery in the groin.

Notes

*This is not the case unfortunately with **inflammatory aneurysms**, which comprise about 5% of infrarenal AAAs overall; here all of these dissection stages can be considerably more difficult.

Uncommonly, the left renal vein **lies behind the aneurysm—identify these patients preoperatively on CT as great care is required when dissecting down the sides of the neck of the aneurysm or when applying the clamp—injury to a retroaortic left renal vein can be catastrophic.

***It always seems a bit odd that in an aneurysm repair you sacrifice the **inferior mesenteric artery**, but usually it's already occluded by thrombus and its job is being done by collateral vessels from the superior mesenteric artery. Uncommonly, however, it is possible that ischaemic colitis can result so always look at the left colon before closing up.

Summary

- The patient is **supine** under **general anaesthetic**
- **Shave**, **prep** and **drape** the whole of the abdomen and groins
- Make either a **midline** or **transverse** incision and perform a full laparotomy
- **Deliver the small bowel** out to the right and wrap in moist swabs and a bag or **pack** in the abdomen
- Follow the **mesentery to its base**
- Insert **Omnitract**
- **Incise peritoneum longitudinally over sac**
- **Dissect duodenum** off the aneurysm neck
- Dissect around the **aneurysm neck**
- Dissect around the **common iliac arteries**
- **Prepare clamps** and give intravenous **heparin**
- **Apply clamps**
- **Open aneurysm sac**
- **Under-run lumbar arteries**
- **Shape the neck** and **iliacs** for anastomosis
- **Size the graft**
- **Suture** in the **neck and test**
- Anastomose the draft distally to either the distal aorta or each common iliac
- Before completing, back bleed and flush
- Let legs back in slowly
- Close peritoneum over graft

13 Below Knee Amputation

Matt Stephenson and Mike Brooks

> **Video** | **22 min 15 s**
> Mike Brooks, Consultant Vascular Surgeon
> Royal Sussex County Hospital, Brighton

Introduction

Allegedly, in the battlefields of the Napoleonic wars, the field medic could cut off an offending limb in a few seconds flat. There would have been little choice in the midst of battle but to do a quick chop and run, or hobble. Unfortunately, such anecdotes are popular with bosses and theatre staff when they feel you're taking too long over a 'simple operation'. Of course, many of those soldiers died of gangrene and very few would have walked.

Respect amputations. They are not minor, quick operations. Getting it right first time is crucial for these often very-high-risk patients. You want a stump that heals, doesn't get infected and for those who will ambulate, will fit a prosthesis. In common usage today, major lower limb amputations are below knee, through knee (coming back into fashion) and above knee. Here we'll demonstrate a below knee amputation, probably the most complex of the three. The two most popular techniques are the long posterior **Burgess flap** and the **skew flap**. Although a Cochrane study showed no difference between the two in terms of healing, the skew flap is favoured by most prosthetists. It creates a less bulbous stump.

Procedure

With the patient under **spinal, epidural** or **general anaesthetic**, **prep** the whole leg except for the foot which you can isolate in a sterile bag (leave any dressings/bandages on the foot—removing them will only release infections). **Drape** to the groin.

Marking the skin flaps accurately is crucial. Take a ruler and mark about **10–12 cm below the femorotibial** joint line. Then make a **circumferential line**

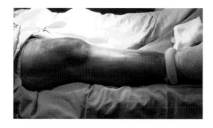
The right leg has been prepped and draped; note the foot is covered with a drape and stockinette.

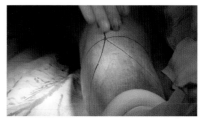
The medial and lateral flaps have been marked; note they are skewed by 2 cm.

around the leg at this level. This will be the level of **tibial transection**. Now measure and make a mark **2 cm lateral to the anterior border** of the tibia (call it **Point A**) along this line. Draw a **straight line** 2 cm long running proximally from point A. Take a **nylon tape** and gently wrap it around the leg at the level of your circumferential line—cut off any redundant tape. The nylon tape length **now equals the leg circumference**, so cut it in two halves. Lay your halved nylon tape around your circumferential line starting at point A, and make a second mark, **point B**, halfway around the leg. **Now halve the tape again** so that it's a quarter of the circumference. Use it to mark a point **halfway between points A and B** on the anteromedial side of the leg. This is **Point C**. Put the quartered Nylon tape running down the leg starting at Point C and mark this—**the apex of the first skin flap**. Keeping it anchored at Point C, swing it round like a compass and mark two or three other points—join these together making a **smooth semicircle**. Repeat on the other side of the leg. Hey

presto—we have now marked our **equal anteromedial and posterolateral** skin flaps. So what was that extra 2-cm line for earlier on? This is an important extension of the incision proximally which allows you to retract the flaps proximally without damaging them to create a sloping bevel on the front of the tibia and successfully divide the fibula at a higher level. Practise all this marking-out on yourself or a friend (but don't proceed any further).

Now **raise your skin flaps**. Make an incision through **skin** and **superficial fascia** straight down and remaining perpendicular to the skin (the incised skin has a tendency to retract up proximally—keep dividing the fascia at the level of the skin flap). Do this all the way around the leg, there will be some sizable superficial vessels, like the long saphenous vein, to tie off. Next incise **through deep fascia** all the way around the leg so muscle is visible. Through a process mainly of blunt dissection **separate this** skin to deep fascia layer **off the underlying muscle** all around the leg. Over the tibia, clearly there is no muscle as it's subcutaneous—here

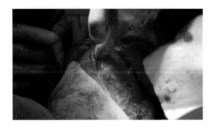

The skin flaps have been raised and retracted up, a finger is bluntly dissecting between the tibia and the anterior compartment muscles to isolate them for division.

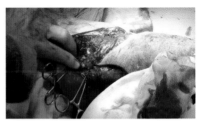

Looking from the lateral aspect. The muscles in the anterior compartment have been divided and the front of the tibia and fibula with intervening interosseus membrane have been dissected. Clips are on the anterior tibial vessels.

you may need sharp dissection to lift it off the periosteum. By the end of this stage you have two equal skin flaps to the depth of fascia that are freed up to the level of your circumferential line—the level of tibial transection.

Next, you need to divide the muscles of the anterior compartments. Starting from the tibia **divide all the muscles of the anterior compartment**, which lie over the fibula and the muscles of the lateral compartment, and tie off the **anterior tibial vessels**. Cut though all these muscles so you come down to see bone all the way around the fronts and sides of the tibia and fibula—you do not need to keep these muscles, they are not important for the skin flap. Then use a **periosteal elevator** to clear the fronts and sides of the tibia and fibula up to the level of tibial transection and 2.5 cm higher on the fibula, which to a certain extent has to be done blindly; it can also be quite oozy. **Transect the fibula 2.5 cm higher** than the tibia with a sharp

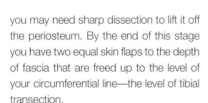

The bone cutter has been passed high up under the skin away from direct vision to transect the fibula high.

double-action bone cutter. Some people use a Gigli saw for this as it's less likely to splinter the bone, but it's more difficult to protect the skin edges from damage.

Then **divide the tibia** at the level of the circumferential line with a saw or a Gigli (be careful—hold the skin flap the way it lay before it retracted up to get an accurate level, also be careful not to catch the skin flaps with the saw—treat those skin flaps reverently). The anterior edge must be **bevelled** by about 1.5 cm and the edges **filed smooth**. The bones are **now separated** and the leg becomes

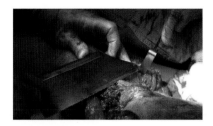

The saw first cuts at 45 degrees to bevel the edge.

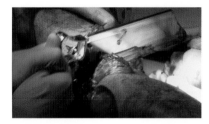

The saw is then turned to perpendicular with the tibia.

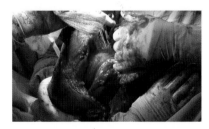

Looking from the medial side. The fibula is being used as a lever to pull the leg forward, stretching the posterior compartment muscles and vessels into view.

floppy allowing access between the two tibial ends to the deep muscles of the leg and the main tibial vessels and nerve—**divide all of these**—tying off the vessels.

For the **nerve** pull this down firmly and separate off any surrounding tissues (there's often a feeding vessel to diathermy), cut it as high as possible and allow it to retract up away into the wound. All that stands in the way of getting that leg into the bin is the **superficial** part of the **posterior compartment**, which comprises the superficial **gastrocnemius** and the deeper bulkier **soleus**. **Retain gastrocnemius—this will be your muscle flap**. You can separate between soleus and gastrocnemius by **blunt dissection** of the fascial layer between them from the medial side and this is best done before division of the bone. Retain gastrocnemius (you'll recognise it by seeing that long strip of plantaris on its deep surface). You'll need a long flap of gastrocnemius and its tendon so it's always worth mobilising some skin off it distally when you're initially cutting the skin flaps. Completely divide all remaining muscle fibres. Put the leg in a labelled sack for incineration.

Now pay attention to ensuring **haemostasis**, excising any **ragged tissue**

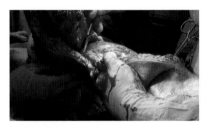

The gastrocnemius is divided low, close to the Achilles tendon—this will be the muscle flap.

and that the bone ends are **smooth**. Leave ligated pedicles and ligatures short so there's minimal tissue to necrose or act as a foreign body. **Irrigate the wound** with copious normal saline to remove any bony fragments that may act as a nidus for infection. **Wrap gastrocnemius** around the tibial stump and **stitch it** to the periosteum over the anterior tibia with several interrupted Vicryl 1 sutures. Now place a **suction drain** deep to this muscle and bring out the drain laterally above the skin flap. Do a continuous layer of absorbable suture such as Vicryl 2–0 **closing the fat/fascial layers** of the two flaps. **Close the skin** with subcuticular absorbable suture. Place Steristrips longitudinally, a dry dressing and stump bandage.

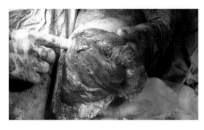

The posterior muscle flap, which is gastrocnemius, has been sutured to the periosteum on the front of the tibia.

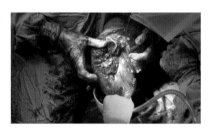

The leg is off. The wound is vigorously irrigated with normal saline to remove clots and bone fragments.

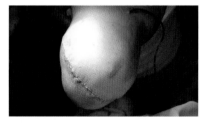

The final stump. The skin has been closed with a subcuticular suture left long at both ends with no knot, with those ends tied loosely together, allowing for swelling of the stump.

Summary

- **Prep** the leg with the foot in a bag and drape to the groin
- **Mark** the anteromedial and posterolateral **skin flaps**
- **Incise** through skin, superficial fascia and deep fascia
- By blunt and sharp dissection **free up** the skin flaps to the circumferential line
- **Divide** the anterior and lateral **muscle groups** and **tie off** the anterior vessels
- Use the **periosteal elevator**

- **Transect** the **fibula** and then the **tibia** (bevel the edge), the fibula **2.5 cm higher**; file smooth.
- **Divide** the **deep posterior muscles**, **tie off** the vessels and **divide the nerve** high
- **Separate soleus and gastrocnemius**, salvaging the latter, sacrificing the former
- Put the leg in the bin
- **Washout**, and **haemostase**
- **Stitch gastrocnemius** to anterior periosteum
- Insert suction **drain**
- **Close** superficial fascia
- **Close** skin subcutaneously
- Steristrips, dry dressing and stump bandage

14 Carotid Endarterectomy

Matt Stephenson and Syed Wacquar Yusuf

> **Video** | **15 min 18 s**
> Syed Wacquar Yusuf, Consultant Vascular
> and Endovascular Surgeon
> Royal Sussex County Hospital, Brighton

Introduction

As surgeons we don't usually have to worry too much about stroke—it's a medical condition isn't it? There's not much we can do surgically for those who have had a **haemorrhagic stroke**, but out of those who have suffered an **ischaemic stroke**, a proportion may have resulted from emboli. Those **emboli** must have come from somewhere, namely either the **heart** or the **extracranial arteries**: the **common** or **internal carotid artery**, or rarely from deep veins (paradoxical embolism in the presence of a patent foramen ovale). That's where we as surgeons can help.

So why does atherosclerotic disease in the carotid cause a stroke? It is mainly due to thrombus forming on the plaque or fragments of that atherosclerotic plaque breaking off and flying up into the brain that causes stroke. Rarely, the reduced flow due to severe narrowing can lead to haemodynamic stroke, particularly if the disease is bilateral and there is additional small vessel disease, and a period of hypotension.

So how are we to know **which patients** who have had a stroke or transient ischaemic attack (TIA) should be treated with a carotid endarterectomy (by the way that simply means opening the artery and **shelling out the plaque** along with the **media** and **intima** of the vessel leaving the adventitia)? People who have strokes often tend to have atherosclerotic disease and some of it is likely to be in the carotid anyway. So, everyone? Carotid artery surgery carries small but significant risks; you need to choose which patients have a greater balance of benefit compared to risk.

How to Operate: for MRCS Candidates and Surgical Trainees, First Edition. M. Stephenson. © 2011 John Wiley & Sons, Ltd.
Published 2011 by John Wiley & Sons, Ltd.

This is where we have to rely on evidence mainly from two big trials: the **North American Symptomatic Carotid Endarterectomy Trial** (NASCET) and the **European Carotid Surgery Trial** (ECST). The bottom line is patients who have had a non-disabling **stroke** or **TIA** with a stenosis in their **internal** or **common carotid artery**, causing a stenosis of **70–99%** on the **affected side** of the brain, should be considered for endarterectomy. You only need to operate on six patients to prevent a stroke if the stenosis is greater than 70%. Patients who have made a good recovery from stroke and have severe stenosis are also considered for surgery, to prevent a more severe event that could be severely disabling or fatal. A completely blocked artery (i.e. 100%) will not allow any flow through it to carry emboli up to the brain anyway. People who have had a dense stroke won't benefit as there's nothing else left to lose neurologically. Stenosis of the external carotid usually does not matter.

One of the biggest subjects of debate in carotid artery surgery is whether to do the operation under **local anaesthetic** (with the patient awake) or under **general anaesthetic**. This operation is going to involve clamping off the blood flow through the internal carotid artery for a while. In most patients, you can get away with this as they will have sufficient blood flow from the vertebral arteries and the contralateral carotid via communicating arteries in the circle of Willis. If not however, within seconds of clamping off the internal carotid, the brain will develop symptoms and signs of ischaemia—if they're awake that is, otherwise you'll only know about it after they've woken from their anaesthetic. That's the benefit of doing the operation awake. You can test whether their brain is dependent on that internal carotid by transiently occluding the vessel with a clamp before opening it and waiting a few minutes or so whilst checking cerebral function by asking questions and giving commands etc. If they don't develop signs of ischaemia, you can proceed with the operation knowing the blood supply to the brain is not compromised and there is no risk of ischaemic injury to the brain (remember brain cells are very susceptible to lack of blood supply and can suffer damage even with a very short period of ischaemia). If they do develop signs of ischaemia, you can prepare to rapidly put in a **shunt** going from the common into the internal carotid artery as soon as you've opened the artery.

If they're asleep, you either have to shunt everyone just in case, or you need to monitor cerebral blood flow using, for instance **trans cranial Doppler** (TCD) flow measurements—using an ultrasound probe over the thinnest part of the temporal bone to detect cerebral flow (not everyone has thin enough bone here—called a TCD window). Alternatively, near infrared spectroscopy can be used for monitoring the mixed oxygen saturation in the cerebral hemispheres.

Lastly, the final thing we know from good evidence is that these operations need to be done **urgently**. The operation should be done within **2 weeks** of the ischaemic event at most to get any benefit from it. Ideally, it should be done within **48 hours**. This is changing the very practice of many vascular departments as priorities are shifting in order to clear out these unstable plaques before they cause a more significant event, that is a stroke or blindness.

Well that was rather a lot of theory for this practical book, and we haven't even got onto the whole patch versus primary closure debate, endarterectomy versus stenting debate, retrojugular approach versus anteromedial approach . . . We'll discuss here a standard approach to the procedure under local anaesthetic.

Procedure

Positioning the patient right is very important; you want to open up the neck as much as possible as well as drain the veins in the neck. So have the patient in the **reverse Trendelenburg** position and put the head in a **head ring** with the **neck slightly extended** and the head **turned away** form you. When this procedure is being carried out under local anaesthesia, it is important to make sure that the patient is comfortable and will be able to stay in that position for up to 2 hours or more. **Prepare** and **drape** the neck and make a **mark** over where your incision will lie. It is best to mark the line of

incision with the neck flexed to take the advantage of the creases for a more cosmetic scar. It is usually done in the anaesthetic room so that the anaesthetist can use it for the superficial infiltration of the local anaesthesia in addition to the cervical block.

The relevant landmarks are the **sternal notch**, the **mastoid** and the **angle of the mandible**. The **sternocleidomastoid muscle** runs between the first of these two and it's along the **anterior border** of this muscle you want to incise. The angle of the mandible is important because you want to stay well clear of it, at least a fingerbreadth in fact, as otherwise you risk damaging the **marginal branch of the mandibular nerve** (a branch of the facial nerve), which would result in an ipsilateral

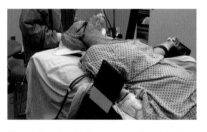

The patient is in the reverse Trendelenburg position with the head in a ring, the cervical spine extended and the head turned away.

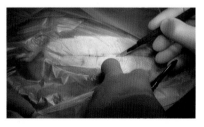

The skin is marked and incised as described.

mouth droop as it supplies part of the orbicularis oris. So, for this reason, many people **curve** the incision slightly posteriorly at the upper part of the sternocleidomastoid.

Check the local anaesthetic block is working by pinching the skin with toothed forceps. **Make an incision** through **skin** and **subcutaneous fat** and you'll then find the **platysma layer**, which is a thin layer of muscle that helps control facial expression. **Cut** straight through it. The next thing to identify is the **sternocleidomastoid** muscle (this stage of dissection is best done with the diathermy blade to minimise bleeding as patients are receiving antiplatelet therapy and the blood supply to the tissues is very good in the neck). Keep dissecting **close to the anterior edge** of it, **retracting this laterally**. You then find yourself on a layer of fascia—the **carotid sheath**—in there lies the common **carotid artery**, the **internal jugular vein** and behind them the **vagus nerve**. **Open this sheath** with forceps

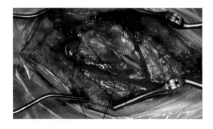

Skin, superficial fascia and platysma has been divided, the sternocleidomastoid is in the lower part of the picture. The facial vein has been ligated.

and scissors. It generally helps to have your assistant retract one edge with forceps and you retract the other with forceps. The first structure you'll find on entering the sheath is the internal jugular vein—a big blue soft structure. Joining this will be one or two tributaries, usually at right angles. The larger of these is the **facial vein**. In the standard approach you **ligate and divide it**. This makes it more mobile to retract the jugular vein laterally to reveal the common carotid artery.

Inserting one or two **self-retaining retractors** is usually quite helpful, with gentle retraction with **Langenbeck** retractors at each end of the wound as you're developing the dissection. Try to get down to the artery itself as soon as you can. You want to stay in the plane directly around the artery—the **periadventitial plane**. Firstly, this is the easiest plane to dissect in, this is loose areolar tissue—God's gift to surgeons. Secondly, it minimises the risk of damage to the vagus nerve which can get injured by the dissection (if the patient is awake it will result in an unpleasant vasovagal experience for the patient, and consequently surgeon). It helps to **infiltrate some more local** anaesthetic at this stage, into the periadventitial tissue, as some patients feel this stage of dissection. Develop the dissection around the common carotid and use right-angled forceps like **Lahey's** to get a **silastic sling** around it. Remember why you're doing this operation—there is potentially **fragile plaque** sitting in that artery—whenever dissecting the carotid, be as careful as you can to not dislodge any further plaque. Dissect the patient off the carotid, not vice versa. The carotid should stay pretty still. **Continue the dissection** superiorly towards the bifurcation but it is important not to dissect the carotid bulb and disturb the plaque at this stage. Another infiltration of plain lignocaine here into the region of the bifurcation is sensible—this theoretically anaesthetises the carotid body, which if over manipulated can result in excessive vagal stimulation.

Next dissect around the distal **internal carotid artery**, again avoid disturbing the carotid bifurcation at this stage. Ask the anaesthetist to administer a bolus of 3000–5000 units of unfractionated heparin and clamp the distal internal and proximal common carotid arteries. Assess the neurological effects of the clamp over the next few minutes. In most cases the collateral circulation is adequate and the patient will not show any features of cerebral ischaemia. Proceed with dissection of the external carotid artery and dissect out the carotid bulb/bifurcation without the risk of embolisation to the brain as the internal carotid artery is clamped. Get a Mixter clamp around the external and **sling** it too. A small bulldog, Ligaclip or ligature will need to be applied to the superior thyroid artery, as this is the first branch of external carotid artery and arises so proximal that it lies below the clamp on the external carotid artery.

How far up should you go with your dissection? How far proximal? You need to dissect up to **normal artery** so that your clamp won't crush the plaque, and you will be able to remove the plaque entirely and repair the artery. You also need sufficient room to insert a shunt on the rare occasion when this may become necessary. How do you know it's normal? Arteries, you will have noticed by now, are not red tubes like in the books. They are white, quite shiny vessels, often with a slightly bluish hue. Atherosclerotic plaques are yellow and you can often see this through the vessel wall. One **gentle squeeze** with atraumatic forceps should be enough to see that the vessel is squishy, not hard. Sometimes this means dissecting up quite high in the neck.

Here you need to be very careful of the **hypoglossal nerve** which hangs down under the angle of the mandible. Damage to the nerve with dissection or diathermy should be avoided by careful dissection. As shown in this case, a branch of the occipital branch of the external carotid artery hooks over the hypoglossal nerve.

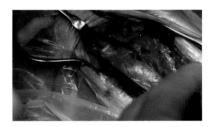

The hypoglossal nerve is hanging down in the way of the dissection. In order to retract it safely superiorly, the occipital artery needs to be ligated and divided.

This branch needs to be divided carefully to allow mobilisation of the hypoglossal nerve for adequate exposure of the distal internal carotid artery.

Which one is the external and which is the internal? The **internal has no branches**, so if there's a branch coming off it, which there should be—the **superior thyroid artery**—it's the external.

A shunt should be readily available for this operation. Rarely, insertion of the shunt may be required if the patient shows features of cerebral hypoxia (under local anaesthesia) or there is a significant change in the middle cerebral flow on TCD monitoring, or there is a significant droop in the mixed oxygen saturation on near infrared spectroscopy. The details of this vary depending on the shunt, but essentially they all consist of a tube that does a loop-the-loop, one end inserts proximally, the other distally. Some have separate channels to blow up balloons to occlude the vessel. A popular choice is the Javid shunt, another one is the Pruit shunt. Make sure you, your assistant and scrub person knows exactly how they work, because if you have to put it in, you have very little time to do it.

Once you are happy that there are no signs of cerebral hypoxia, make a longitudinal arteriotomy over the soft, disease-free part of the common carotid artery using an **11 blade** and extend the arteriotomy with **Potts scissors** extending across the carotid bulb into the internal carotid artery until you have 'healthy'

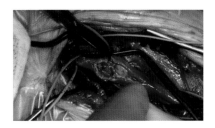

The artery has been opened to reveal the plaque.

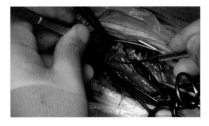

The Watson–Cheyne dissector is gently lifting off the plaque.

artery each side of the plaque. Use a **Watson-Cheyne dissector** to dissect between the plaque and the arterial wall, which is left very thin, really just adventitia. Dissect it off in both directions. It often helps to get a **MacDonald dissector** round the back of it, between plaque and carotid wall, and then cut down with a knife onto the dissector—this allows you to lift the leading edge of the plaque away from the vessel wall. Make sure there are no little strands of tissue that might fly off into the brain later that night. **Irrigate** the inside with heparinised saline.

Some surgeons then **close the arteriotomy** primarily using 7–0 Prolene suture. This should be done with due

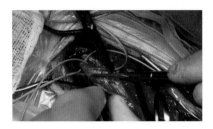

The cleaned out artery—a final check is made for any loose strands that could embolise.

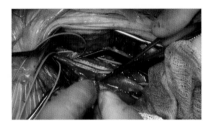

The synthetic patch is sutured into place to prevent narrowing of the vessels secondary to the arteriotomy.

care without narrowing the artery. However, if there is any concern about narrowing then it is safer to close the arteriotomy with a synthetic patch. The majority of surgeons, however, tend to use a patch as it can compensate for the slightly narrowing effect suturing the edges together can have. Others always use a patch. Before finally tying the knot, allow some **back bleeding** from the internal and external carotid and a little in flow from the common carotid to clear these of any clot that may have formed, and then **flush** them with heparinised saline. Finally **tie** the knot. Gently **remove** the external carotid clamp and then the common carotid clamp. Finally, the internal carotid clamp is removed after a few heartbeats. This sequence is used to divert any debris or clot towards the external carotid artery as the consequences of any emboli going up the external carotid artery are likely to be insignificant. Check for bleeding; a little ooze from the anastomosis line usually stops with patience and gentle pressure with a swab. Check for remaining **haemostasis** on the way out. Most people insert a **suction drain** as a haematoma in the neck could lead to problems with airways.

Close the platysma with an absorbable suture such as 2–0 Vicryl, then the **skin** with another continuous absorbable suture like Monocryl 3–0.

Summary

- **Position** the patient to fully expose the operative site
- **Prep** and **drape**
- Incise through **skin**, subcutaneous **fat** and **platysma with a diathermy blade**
- Identify **sternocleidomastoid** and **retract it laterally**
- **Open the carotid sheath**
- Ligate and divide the **facial vein**
- **Retract the internal jugular vein** laterally

- Reinfiltrate with **plain lignocaine**
- Dissect the **common carotid** and **sling** this
- Dissect the distal **internal carotid** and **sling** it
- Give **IV heparin** and **wait** 3 minutes
- **Dissect the external carotid and sling it**
- **Clamp** the arteries starting with the internal

- Perform an **arteriotomy**
- Insert **shunt** if necessary
- Perform **endarterectomy**
- **Irrigate**
- Partially close **primarily** or with **patch**
- Allow **back bleeding** and **flush**
- **Close arteriotomy** fully
- Check for **haemostasis** and insert suction **drain**
- **Close platysma** and **skin**

15 Temporal Artery Biopsy

Matt Stephenson and Utham R Shanker

> **Video** | **3 min 33 s**
> Utham R Shanker, Consultant
> Eastbourne District General Hospital, Eastbourne

Introduction

When the physicians suspect **giant cell arteritis** they need us to provide the histopathologists with a small segment of temporal artery for diagnosis. Ideally, this needs to be done as soon as possible after making the clinical diagnosis, as they will have started high-dose steroids empirically and should be within a week of starting steroids. With each passing day, the steroid treatment may therefore result in **false-negative** results (although starting steroids shouldn't be delayed in cases of high suspicion). In some trusts they are slotted into dedicated spaces on minor op lists. In others they fit into CEPOD lists or on the end of elective lists. Either way, temporal artery biopsy is a neat little operation which doesn't take long to learn.

Bear in mind it must be rather peculiar having an operation on your face whilst you're awake. Maxillofacial surgeons must deal with this all the time. Do try to keep up a pleasant conversation with the patient.

Procedure

During your preoperative discussion with the patient you must **mark the temporal artery**. This is in fact the most important thing about this operation. Marking it inaccurately or marking where you could actually feel the pulsation in your own fingers will result in you not being able to find the artery, which would be terribly embarrassing. If the artery is very diseased, often all you can feel is a **hard cord** running where the pulsation should be—mark this instead. If you can't find the artery at all on the symptomatic side, try the other side. If you can't find one at all (very unusual) don't proceed. Blindly digging around in the hope of finding a non-pulsatile, non-cord like temporal

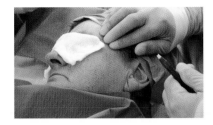

Palpating the pulsation carefully.

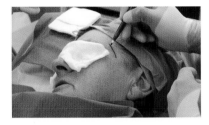

A very accurate mark being drawn.

is very relaxing for the patient, protects their eyes from the theatre lights and helps maintain field sterility.

Inject some **local anaesthetic** (lignocaine 1% or whatever you fancy) into the skin and subcutaneous tissues under your mark. **Recheck** one last time that your mark is exactly over the artery. Make an **incision** exactly over the middle of your mark. It needs to be about **2 cm** or so. **Deepen** through **skin, subcutaneous fat** and **superficial fascia**. Keep feeling the artery intermittently to check it's right underneath. There may be a layer of **obvious fascia** to divide and then you're on to the artery. Sometimes, however, it is remarkably superficial—try not to cut straight into the artery. Swap for dissecting scissors and forceps and gradually **dissect** out the artery. Opening and closing the jaws of a haemostatic clip is a useful way of opening up the space. There may be some **branches**, each of which can be **ligated** and **divided**. Make sure it's not vein you're taking, they can look similar. Get a **tie** around **each end** of the main artery and then **cut out** the segment between the ties. You want at

artery would be ill advised. In terms of landmarks, it's usually around two fingerbreadths above the zygomatic arch.

With the patient **comfortable** and **supine** and the **head turned** slightly away from you, **recheck** that the mark is accurate before prepping; reapply some marker pen if needed. **Prep** the temporal area as far as the lateral edge of the eyebrow and gently stroke the hair moistened by prep back away from the area. Some people **shave** a small patch of skin so that the incision can be placed behind the hairline. Put two **square drapes** to cover the hair, leaving the face undraped. Ask the patient to **close their eyes** and lay a **moistened gauze swab** over them. This

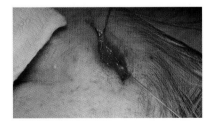

Both ends of the artery have been ligated.

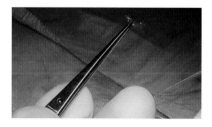

The specimen. They shrink as soon as they removed, which always make them look quite underwhelming.

least **1 cm** of artery, more if you can. Bear in mind it shrivels up as soon as you remove it and can look most unimpressive. **Stop any bleeding** and close the skin with **subcuticular** absorbable suture such as 3–0 Monocryl, or interrupted sutures as seen in this video. You can use a spray on **op site dressing** so you don't have the awkwardness of applying a sticky dressing to hair.

Summary

- **Mark** the temporal artery very accurately
- **Prep** and **drape**, covering the **eyes** with a **swab**
- **Inject** local anaesthetic
- **Incise** down through skin, fat and fascia
- **Dissect** out the artery with scissors and forceps
- **Ligate** and **divide** all branches
- **Ligate** both ends and **excise segment** of temporal artery at least 1 cm long
- Send to **histopathology**
- **Haemostase** and **close** the skin

16 Femorodistal Bypass

Matt Stephenson and Karim El-Sakka

> **Video** | **14 min 43 s**
> Karim El-Sakka, Consultant Vascular Surgeon
> Royal Sussex County Hospital, Brighton

Introduction

One of the 'big three' index operations in vascular surgery along with the abdominal aortic aneurysm and the carotid endarterectomy, this is the core of vascular surgical practice and can take anything from 2 hours to all day. This operation requires skills in careful preoperative **case selection**, **dissection**, **fine anastomoses** and **patience**. The results, however, can be truly worth the effort, considering 5-year patency rates stand at around 70%. The two indications for a femorodistal anastomosis are: (1) **critical limb ischaemia** and (2) **severe intermittent claudication**, where other treatments have failed. There isn't space here to go into more detail of the whys and wherefores but essentially this operation is about plumbing a graft from the common or superficial femoral artery to whichever vessel is patent further down. Which vessel to plumb onto is determined by preoperative imaging using some combination of duplex scanning, magnetic resonance angiography (MRA), computed tomography angiography (CTA) or digital subtraction angiography (DSA).

So, essentially you need a good vessel to plumb into at the top (i.e. **good inflow** so relatively non-diseased aorta and iliac), a **good conduit**, ideally being the ipsilateral long saphenous vein (or less preferably a polytetrafluoroethylene (PTFE) graft with lower long-term patency and higher infection risk), and a good vessel to plumb on to which isn't blocked further down (i.e. **good run-off**). The aim of the operation is to improve blood flow to the foot so that ulcers can heal or your patient can get back to playing golf.

Procedure

Prior to the procedure the patient has been to the vascular laboratory to have the **long saphenous vein marked** along its length to aid identification for harvest. If the distal artery that is to be anastomosed is very distal and therefore superficial, it can also be **marked** for ease of identification. The patient is **supine** under **general anaesthetic** or **epidural**, the groin is

How to Operate: for MRCS Candidates and Surgical Trainees, First Edition. M. Stephenson. © 2011 John Wiley & Sons, Ltd.
Published 2011 by John Wiley & Sons, Ltd.

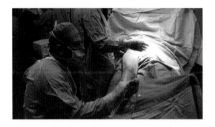

One surgeon usually sits at the site of distal dissection, the other stands at the groin.

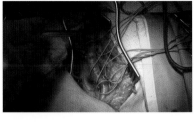

The common, profunda and superficial femoral arteries, including all the branches have been slung with silastic slings.

shaved and the leg **prepped** down to the foot, which is placed in a **sterile transparent bag**, and a **U-shaped drape** covers from above the groin.

One surgeon starts the dissection of the groin to find the femoral artery whilst the other surgeon starts the dissection of the distal vessel. And so begins the **race**. Although of course it's not a race, it's all done very carefully and methodically.

The groin dissection begins with an **oblique incision** over the femoral artery, which should be pulsatile if you're doing the correct operation (if it's not pulsatile there'll be no inflow). The incision should start **just above the inguinal ligament** (use the bony landmarks of the pubic tubercle and anterior superior iliac spine (ASIS) to help, not the visible groin crease as with age and obesity the latter descends considerably compared to the former) and course **inferomedially**, obliquely over the femoral artery so that it can be extended over the course of the long saphenous vein. Dissect down through **superficial fascia** and **fat**, being guided towards the pulsating femoral

artery. Stay on the **lateral side** of the artery, pushing the tissue medially thus avoiding excessive injury to **lymphatic tissue**. Dissect down on to the common femoral artery at the level just below the inguinal ligament. Dissect all around the artery keeping close to it, that is in the **periadventitial plane**. Aim to get a silastic **sling** around it early, using right-angled forceps like **Lahey's** so that you can gently pull it up and **control it** to help with further dissection. Note the **calibre of the vessel changes** a few centimetres from the inguinal ligament; this is because it has **bifurcated** and the **profunda** has branched off behind. Gently dissect inferior to the femoral bifurcation and get a sling around the **superficial femoral artery**. Gently lift up on the two slings and the profunda will appear coming off behind. **Double sling this**. **Dissect** out all the **branches**. Double **sling** all the **branches**.

The **distal dissection** depends entirely on which vessel you're plumbing on to. If it has been marked by preoperative duplex it's very easy, just keep dissecting down

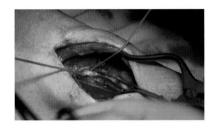

The distal vessel has been dissected out, and slings placed around it proximally and distally.

and soon enough you'll come to said vessel. Just like with the groin, dissect out the vessel; there may be **venae comitantes** around it. Get a **sling** around it at one end and then another sling at the other, and check that the artery is **soft** and **compressible**. More likely you may, however, have no such mark and you are aiming instead for the distal popliteal (in which case this is a fem-pop bypass) or one of the trifurcated branches. The following is how you get to each:

1 **Popliteal**—for the above knee popliteal, palpate the femoral shaft on the medial surface of the thigh and feel the groove behind that. Make a longitudinal incision over this, corresponding to the anterior border of the sartorius. Deepen the incision and retract the sartorius posteriorly revealing the popliteal fat pad, within which is the neurovascular bundle. The artery is surrounded by a plexus of veins. For the below-knee popliteal, make an incision on the medial aspect of the calf along the border of gastrocnemius. Deepen the incision and dissect between the medial head of the muscle and the tibia. Lift the vein away to expose the popliteal artery.

The **infrageniculate vessels**—namely the anterior tibial, posterior tibial and the peroneal; in addition to using the above approach for the infrageniculate popliteal artery, you can continue the dissection inferiorly by dividing the soleus off the back of the tibia. You can then follow the popliteal artery down to its bifurcation into anterior tibial and tibioperoneal trunk. You can access the first 1.5 cm of the anterior tibial and the proximal peroneal and posterior tibial from here, but for those arteries when they become more distal, read on:

2 **Anterior tibial**—make a vertical incision in the anterolateral aspect of the leg about 1 cm lateral to the tibial crest. Deepen to between the anterior tibial tendon medially and the extensor hallucis longus tendon laterally, which is retracted laterally.

3 **Posterior tibial**—make a vertical incision of about 10 cm along the medial edge of the Achilles tendon. Deepen to separate the fused gastrocnemius and soleus posteriorly and the flexor digitorum longus anteriorly.

4 **Peroneal**—to access the proximal peroneal, it's usually easier to approach it from the medial incision described above for the infrageniculate popliteal artery but for the distal peroneal a lateral incision on the leg is needed with resection of a short segment of fibula.

Whoever finishes their dissection has the reward of starting to **harvest the long saphenous vein**. Finding it is easy when it's been preoperatively marked by duplex. Just remember it's sometimes very superficial so don't go and cut right through it after opening the skin! Try to leave a **bridge of skin** between the groin dissection and the long saphenous vein harvest. **Dissect out the vein** and **ligate** and **divide** all the tributaries the whole length of the vein. Tie them well because shortly that low pressure vein is about to have arterial pressure through it, hopefully. Ligate it distally as low as possible checking you'll have enough length to get to the distal artery. Don't completely divide it yet. Make a small **venotomy** and **flush** heparinised saline up it. Firstly, it's to **flush** it of thrombus and, secondly, it's to see if there are any **holes leaking** from ties that were tied badly or other iatrogenic injury. Whilst flushing, squeeze the vein closed with your fingers at ever more proximal intervals so the pressure in the vein is high in that part, thus revealing defects. Repair any such leaky holes and blame your assistant for them. **Ligate** and **divide** it close to the **saphenofemoral**

junction and **distally** when happy it's not going to leak, and put it in a bowl of **heparinised saline**.

Now prepare to do the **proximal anastomosis**. Ask the anaesthetist to kindly give about 5000 units of **intravenous heparin** and 3 minutes later **clamp proximally** on the common femoral artery and **distally** on the **profunda** and **superficial femoral** (the 3 minutes also gives you time to choose your clamps). Make a vertical **arteriotomy**. **Fashion the distal end** of the vein into a **spatulated** shape and perform a standard **vascular anastomosis** of the distal end of the long saphenous vein to the common femoral artery. Flush the vein and briefly release each clamp in turn to back bleed out any thrombus before closing the arteriotomy. Put a soft clamp on the vein. This is therefore a **reversed vein graft**. If you don't reverse it and plumb the top of the vein to the femoral artery, this is an ***in situ* graft**. Both are acceptable. The disadvantage of the *in situ* technique is that you need to destroy the valves in the vein with a **valvulotome**, which can damage the lining of the vein. It does, however, have the advantage that you're plumbing similarly sized vein and artery together, which is technically less challenging.

You need to create a **tunnel** for your new bypass to pass through. This broadly speaking can be **subcutaneous** or **subfascial**. For the former, take the long curvy sharp tunneller and pass it from above down or below up feeling it pass

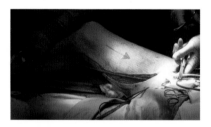

A long incision has been made up the length of the long saphenous vein, which has then been dissected out.

under the skin and poke out the other hole. **Take care**. Tie a **thread** to one end of it and pull that through your tunnel, so there's only a thread going through the tunnel now. Tie the **other end of the vein to the thread** coming out of the groin wound and pull on the other end of the thread from below, thus passing it through the previously made tunnel. Perform a **vascular anastomosis** distally. These are **titchy vessels** so you will require magnifying **loupes** to see what you're doing. Before completing the anastomosis, **flush** the vein again and distally with heparinised saline.

Release the soft clamp on the vein in the groin. The blood should now be flowing down the common femoral artery in to the reversed long saphenous vein graft and into the outflow vessel. **Check the pulse** distally. Don't expect it to be palpable but do expect at least a **monophasic** signal with your intraoperative Doppler machine—**mark** the skin where you found it so it's easy for nurses doing their obs to

check it later and reduces the chance of you being called at 2 AM because it can't be found. **Close** all the wounds, firstly with absorbable suture such as 2–0 Vicryl to fascia and fat where appropriate and then subcutaneous absorbable suture to skin. If one wound area is a bit oozy, a suction **drain** is appropriate.

Notes

Sometimes the patient no longer has an ipsilateral long saphenous vein as it's been stripped before or long since emigrated to the heart. Or it may be thrombosed or varicose in which case it won't do for a bypass conduit. Look first to the other leg as this is plan B. If this fails, scan the patient's arms and see if their basilic veins are any good (not thrombosed and at least 3 mm diameter). If they really have no decent vein however, then you will have to resort to a synthetic PTFE graft which has a lower long term patency rate and more considerable consequences if it gets infected.

Summary
- Make sure the patient's long saphenous vein has been **marked preoperatively** in the vascular laboratory +/− distal artery
- With the patient under **general anaesthetic** or **epidural**, **prep** and **drape** the leg
- One surgeon performs a standard groin dissection to **expose** and **control the**
- One surgeon performs the distal dissection to **expose** and **control the distal artery**
- **Harvest** the long saphenous vein
- **Flush test** the vein
- Create a **subcutaneous** (or subfascial) **tunnel** using the tunneller and pass a long Vicryl thread through it

(Continued)

- Perform an **anastomosis** of the femoral artery to the distal long saphenous vein
- **Tunnel** the vein
- Perform an **anastomosis** of the distal artery to the proximal long saphenous vein
- **Flush** the vein and distal vessel before closure
- Check for a **Doppler signal**
- **Haemostase** and consider suction **drains**
- **Close** fat/ fascia and skin
- **Dry dressings** to all wounds

17 Brachiocephalic Fistula

Matt Stephenson and Karim El-Sakka

> **Video** | 8 min 5 sec
> Karim El-Sakka, Consultant Vascular Surgeon
> Royal Sussex County Hospital, Brighton

Introduction

With the prevalence of **chronic renal failure** rising and the number of organ donors relatively static, the need to provide a **renal access** service is on the up. **Arteriovenous fistulae** can cause huge amounts of confusion amongst medical students and doctors because they can seem rather mysterious. What is an arteriovenous fistula exactly? It is a fistula created surgically by making a small hole in an artery, finding a nearby vein which you ligate and divide, and plumb on to the hole in the artery thereby directing arterial blood up the vein back to the heart (it can of course also be congenital, traumatic etc.). This has the effect of gradually distending the vein all the way up the limb and 4–6 weeks later you have a broad area of vein to cannulate for haemodialysis.

Fistulae won't necessarily last forever, they **thrombose** or become **aneurysmal** and may then need to be revised. The principles are that you create the primary fistula as **distal as possible** and then move proximally if it fails, so the usual stages are: **radiocephalic** (at the wrist), **brachiocephalic** (antecubital fossa), **brachiobasilic** (antecubital fossa but slightly more complicated) and then, when these fail on both upper limbs, **PTFE grafts** from the brachial artery up to the axillary vein. But there is a lot of variation on this depending on where you work. It does get much more complicated than this in some unfortunate patients.

When cannulating or venesecting renal failure patients always spare them their more proximal veins and keep to the hand as much as possible. Repeated needling of veins causes them to thrombose and this will render the big cephalic and basilic veins unusable for later fistulae, should they need them. Most patients will require a duplex scan of the veins and arms to check arterial size and patency (you usually need at least a

3-mm radial artery for a radiocephalic) and venous patency—a subclavian vein stenosis from previous central venous catheterisation for instance may need to be angioplastied prior to the procedure otherwise they may develop venous hypertension in the limb postoperatively. Some prefer to only anastomose onto veins they can visibly see through the skin in outpatients.

We've shown the brachiocephalic fistula as it's easier to see than a titchy radio-cephalic, and it's widely practised.

Procedure

The patient is **supine** and **awake** with the arm **abducted** and **supinated** on an arm board. The whole upper limb is **prepped** up to the axilla excluding the hand, which is then wrapped in a drape and stockin-ette with an arm drape covering from upper arm and beyond.

Inject **0.5% bupivocaine** into the skin and subcutaneous tissues in a line **1 cm distal and parallel with the elbow flexor crease**. Make a **transverse incision** in the same line, 1 cm distal and parallel with the elbow flexor crease. Deepen the incision through **skin**, **superficial fascia** and **fat** and insert a **self-retaining retractor** such as a West retractor. Using **dissecting scissors** explore the **cubital fossa**, looking for a big vein—it's usually very obvious.

Often the first vein to be found is going transversely, this is probably the **median cubital vein**. Follow it laterally to the large trunk vein on the lateral side of the fossa—the cephalic vein. **Skeletalise** it using careful dissection keeping **close to the vein,** thus keeping in the easiest plane and minimising collateral damage. **Ligate** and **divide the tributaries** until there is a reasonable length of vein to swing around to the artery but don't ligate or divide the vein itself yet—get a silastic sling round it to help control it. Use a **marker pen** on the anterior surface of the vein so you **don't twist it** later when swinging it round.

Next, explore the middle/medial part of the fossa for the **brachial artery** using its

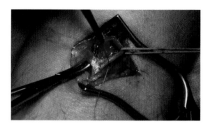

The cephalic vein has been slung laterally and the Lahey forceps have isolated the median cubital vein for ligation and division.

The skin incision.

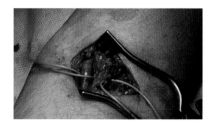

The brachial artery has also been dissected and slung. The anterior surface of the vein has been marked to avoid twisting it.

pulsation to guide you. Unlike the vein it is covered in a definite, clearly seen **bicipital aponeurosis,** which you can **cut through** with scissors. Continue dissecting down to isolate a segment of artery, keeping close to the artery, thus keeping in the right plane and minimising collateral damage. Get a **sling** around it. Always do it in this order, that is explore the **vein first** because if it's not usable, due to thrombosis or size for instance, it avoids unnecessary dissection of the artery.

Using small **bulldog clamps**, clamp **proximally** and **distally** on the brachial artery and make a vertical **arteriotomy** about the length of one-third the circumference of the artery, very slightly lateral to the front of the artery. Use a bulldog clamp proximally on the cephalic vein and **ligate it distally** with an absorbable suture such as 2–0 Vicryl. Make a small **venotomy** at the distal end of the cephalic vein just above the ligature and open out the vein by **cutting proximally** up the vein about the length of the arteriotomy. **Flush** the vein with **heparinised saline**

(thrombosis happens quickly in veins with no flow). So the artery is lying there in the medial side of the fossa and the vein still in the lateral side some way apart. Of course you could just cut the vein now, just above the ligature and swing it round to meet its new friend but trying to stitch a vein that's flapping in the breeze is more difficult than stitching one that's anchored in place. So start the anastomosis with them geographically distant and do a **parachute technique**. Using fine non-absorbable suture such as **7–0 Prolene** go from **in to out on the artery** just lateral to the apex of the arteriotomy and then go through the **vein from out to in** at a corresponding place on the vein. Continue in the same way gradually going round the apex of the arteriotomy and venotomy until all the way around by about three stitches each side. *Now* **cut the vein** just above the ligature and **parachute** it across to the artery by pulling both ends of the suture. **Continue the anastomosis** but before completing and finally tying the knot, **release** the **distal arterial clamp** briefly to let it back bleed and thus remove any thrombus,

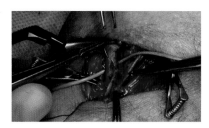

The artery has been opened longitudinally and the vein is being anastomosed to it.

release the **proximal clamp** briefly to check inflow and remove thrombus and **release** the **vein clamp** briefly to remove thrombus and then **flush** it with heparinised saline. Whilst doing this feel that the flush is flushing easily with no impedance. **Complete the anastomosis** and feel over the arm for a **thrill** in the vein.

Always then **explore** around the more proximal cephalic vein as it lies in a **fascial** envelope which can kink it and there may be some bands or tributaries to divide in order to keep it straight and hence working properly. Ensure **haemostasis** and **close just the skin** with absorbable suture such as subcuticular 3–0 Monocryl. The patient can usually go home the same day; advise them to keep the arm straight for the next 24 hours and suggest they might like a nice cup of tea.

Summary

- The patient is **supine** with the arm **abducted** comfortably on an **arm board**
- Inject **local anaesthetic** in a line **1 cm distal** and **parallel** with the elbow **flexor crease**
- **Incise** in the same line
- Identify and dissect out the **cephalic vein**, control with **slings**
- Divide the **bicipital aponeurosis**
- Identify and dissect out the **brachial artery**, control with **slings**
- **Open** the vein, **flush** it and **mark** the anterior surface
- **Clamp** the artery **superiorly** and **inferiorly**
- Perform an **arteriotomy**
- Do a **parachute anastomosis**, dividing the vein before parachuting down
- **Flush** before final tying
- Check for **resistance**
- **Close** the skin with subcuticular absorbable suture

18 Scrotal Exploration

Epididymal Cysts and Orchidectomy

Matt Stephenson and Stephen Whitehead

> **Video** | **11 min 26 s**
> Stephen Whitehead, Consultant General Surgeon
> Conquest Hospital, St Leonards-on-Sea

Introduction

Even if you don't want to be a urologist, it's quite likely you will have to cover urology, at least out of hours, at some time in your surgical career path. Exploring the scrotum is of course one of the most pressing emergencies facing urologists in the scenario of a suspected torsion of the testis. However, that often means the general surgical registrar out of hours in many hospitals. Fortunately, you'll be glad to know that exploring the scrotum isn't rocket science.

There is a standard approach you can use to enter the scrotal sac and deliver out the contents for inspection. Unlike in an exploratory laparotomy, for instance, you usually know quite clearly what to expect before opening up—clinical examination of the scrotum along with ultrasound where necessary are very helpful.

So although these two videos happens to show scrotal exploration followed by excision of epididymal cysts in the first case and orchidectomy in the second, the general principles apply to the other reasons you might want to look inside someone's scrotum and we return to this in the *Notes* section.

Specifically regarding **epididymal cysts**—these are common and in young men who are asymptomatic should generally be left alone. This is because excising them risks sterility of that testis, potentially resulting in reduced fertility. In the elderly gentleman with large swellings in his scrotum that may be uncomfortable and awkward, this is obviously less of a concern. They do unfortunately have a risk of recurrence and it's not uncommon to have a fairly bruised, swollen scrotum postoperatively.

How to Operate: for MRCS Candidates and Surgical Trainees, First Edition. M. Stephenson. © 2011 John Wiley & Sons, Ltd.
Published 2011 by John Wiley & Sons, Ltd.

Always make sure you have carefully examined the scrotum and abdomen pre-operatively so that you're confident about what you're dealing with. Have you excluded a coexistent hernia or even a hernia mimicking a scrotal swelling (**can you get above it?**)? Can you **feel the testis** and does it feel benign? Can you feel the scrotal swelling **separately from the testis** (as in the case of epididymal cysts)?

Procedure

With the patient **supine** under **general anaesthetic**, **shave**, **prep** and **drape** the scrotum. **Cup** the side of the **scrotum** in your hand **stretching the skin** of the anterior surface of the scrotum over the lump (or the testis if that's what you're aiming for). You'll notice the vessels in the skin are running **transversely** so with the skin taut over the lump, make a **transverse incision** between these vessels (not because you're worried you'll cause skin ischaemia; just so it doesn't bleed as much).

Incise through **skin** and then straight through **dartos muscle**. There then seem to be innumerable, very thin layers covering the testis (or lump, whichever you're incising down onto) to incise through. They are in fact the **external**, **middle** and **internal spermatic fasciae**

(and if you were incising straight down on to testis you'd then encounter the **tunica vaginalis**).

They don't come labelled unfortunately, so open each layer **cautiously** until you're on to **cyst wall**. Try your best **not to rupture** it. If you do it's not disastrous, it just makes dissecting it out a lot more difficult. **Deliver it** along with the testis out of the wound. Using a combination of sharp and blunt dissection, **dissect** around the cyst wall down to the neck of the cyst where it emerges from the epididymis and **divide it** there. If there's more than one cyst, obviously repeat for all of them. Often there isn't much left of the epididymis if there have been multiple, large cysts. If doing an orchidectomy, having delivered the testis doubly transfix the cord with a strong absorbable suture such as 0 Vicryl and send to histology as appropriate.

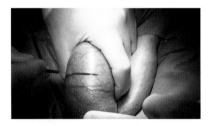

A transverse incision in the right hemiscrotum. The skin needs to be stretched over the underlying lump.

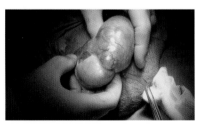

The testis and epididymal cysts have been delivered (the testis is the white structure).

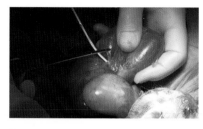

The cyst is held in the non-dominant hand as it is dissected free from the other scrotal contents.

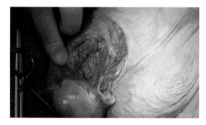

The cysts have been excised. You can see the testis hanging down from the cord structures which have been separated by the large cysts.

Deal with any bleeding points and **return** the scrotal contents back into the scrotum. **Close the dartos** layer with absorbable sutures (important for haemostasis) and then the **skin** with a subcuticular absorbable continuous suture.

Notes

For a suspected **torsion of the testis**, do everything described to get into the scrotum and deliver the contents but obviously your attention will then be on the cord and the testis: **Is the cord twisted**? Does the testis look **blue** or even **black**

(it's **normally white** so pallor isn't a useful sign to report in your op note)? If it's twisted and the testis looks viable untwist it and perform an **orchidopexy**. If it's twisted and the testis has turned blue, **untwist it** and **wrap the testis** in a **warm swab** and **reassess** after several minutes. If it then loses its blue tinge go straight on to the orchidopexy step. If it's twisted and the testis is frankly **black and unsalvageable**, it's best not to untwist it which would allow the ischaemic toxins in to the blood stream—instead **transfix** and **divide the cord**—but do have a very low threshold for giving it a chance and seeing how it looks after the warm swab treatment. If in doubt it's usually better not to do an orchidectomy, return it to the scrotum and make sure the patient has follow up with the urologists.

Of course, in the majority of cases you'll find that the cord is entirely normal and untwisted, the testis is perfectly healthy and you wonder what all the fuss was about at four in the morning, do an orchidopexy anyway, it may have twisted and untwisted. For the orchidopexy, simply stitch the outer layer of the testis (the tunica) to the inside of the scrotum at three points, so that it can no longer twist. Always **repeat** on the other side as a prophylactic measure whether the testis was twisted at the time of surgery or not. For this reason, some people advocate that in the case of suspected torsion of the testes, rather than a transverse incision, a midline incision is best, from which both sides of the scrotum can be accessed.

Summary

- The patient is **supine** under **general anaesthetic**
- **Shave**, **prep** and **drape** the scrotum
- **Stretch the skin** of the scrotum over the lump
- **Incise** through **skin**, **dartos** and **underlying layers**
- **Deliver** the **cyst** and **testis**
- **Dissect** out the cyst
- **Divide** it at the base
- **Repeat** for other cysts
- **Haemostasis**
- **Return contents** to scrotum
- Close **dartos** and **skin**

19 Vasectomy

Matt Stephenson and Vasileios Trompetas

> **Video** | **8 min 34 s**
> Vasileios Trompetas, Consultant General Surgeon
> Eastbourne District General Hospital, Eastbourne

Introduction

The vasectomy is rather unique in this book and DVD in that it is the only procedure you do on someone who actually has nothing pathologically wrong with them other than the ability to make babies. Whereas many patients who do have something wrong with them will accept the odd complication of surgery as a trade-off for getting rid of their pathology, these perfectly healthy patients may find that more of a struggle. That simply means trying to avoid as much discomfort as possible by being generous with the local anaesthetic, being meticulous with antisepsis and haemostasis to reduce the chance of infection and haematoma, and, of course, making certain you have divided and ligated the vas deferens and not a strand of fascia . . . Detailed, standardised counselling and consent is essential to minimise the risks of litigation.

Procedure

With the patient **supine**, legs just **slightly apart** and **genitals** fully **uncovered** firstly **examine** each cord in turn to make sure that you can clearly identify the vas deferens. Firstly, feel the **testes** and check there is no abnormality here (it would be embarrassing to miss a coincidental growth on the testis in this peak risk age group), then **palpate the cord** from epididymis up to the external ring just above the pubic bone and note any cysts on the cord or in the epididymis. Don't want to teach you to suck eggs but the vas is that **firm thick** cord-like structure in the middle of all the other more strandy cord-like structures.

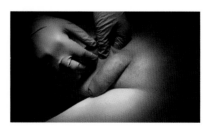

Scrotal examination. The cord is being examined.

How to Operate: for MRCS Candidates and Surgical Trainees, First Edition. M. Stephenson. © 2011 John Wiley & Sons, Ltd.
Published 2011 by John Wiley & Sons, Ltd.

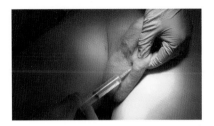

The nerve block.

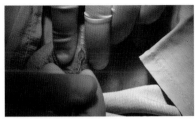

The left hand is holding the vas in three-point fixation and the right hand is incising over it.

Before you prep, inject a **nerve block**. Retract the penis superiorly and insert your needle into the **midline raphe** on the ventral surface of the scrotum. Aim it up towards the external ring on one side and inject 5 ml of **1% lignocaine** in the region of the cord, and repeat on the other side (you can do all this through one skin prick). Now **shave** and **prep** the genitals and surrounding area, and **drape** just the scrotum.

Next **pick up the vas deferens** on one side between your **thumb** on the posterior side and your **second and third fingers** on the other side of the scrotum, thus making **three-point fixation** of the vas, with the thumb pushing it anteriorly and the fingers each side of it so the vas is stretched out under the skin over your thumb and very superficial under the skin. With your other hand inject 1 ml of 2% lignocaine + adrenaline into the skin directly over the vas. **Wait** for this to work without letting go of the vas.

Maintaining the three-point fixation, make a **small incision** (less than 1 cm) transversely over the palpable vas and **deepen** through the external spermatic

fascial layers. Now use special **vasectomy ringed forceps** to get round the vas and **draw it out**. It's likely there will still be a layer or two of fascia over it, which you can **incise** and then replace the ringed forceps around the vas itself.

Gradually **dissect** out a length of vas deferens from its covering fascia and get **clips on both ends. Cut** in between them. If you left it at this, of course, there's a pretty good chance those sperm are going to eventually find their way back down the two cut ends resulting in further trips to Mothercare so **ligate** the distal end and for the proximal end, **ligate** it but

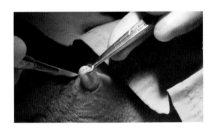

The vas has been delivered and an incision made over its covering fibres.

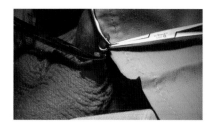

The vas has been divided and each end held in a clip.

also **fold it back on itself** and **doubly ligate** it in the folded back position.

Make sure you've obtained **haemostasis**—bruising is common but significant bleeding and haematoma is rare. Diathermy is generally avoided as it reduces the success rate of reversal of vasectomy; swab pressure usually works, but do remember if essential—only use bipolar given it's on an appendage. Let the two ends drop back inside and **close the skin** with a couple of interrupted absorbable sutures. **Repeat on the other side**.

Advise the patient to wear **tight fitting pants** to begin with to reduce swelling and haematoma risk. Encourage sexual activity to get rid of any existing sperm and ensure the use of an alternative means of **contraception** until a sperm **count** at 16 weeks confirms success. Failure to clear the sperm is rare and requires further sperm counts. If persistent, it is usually the result of duplicate vas deferens on one side, if technical failure is excluded. It requires redo vasectomy under general anaesthetic to allow for exploration of the scrotum. Remember that no form of contraception, including a vasectomy, is 100% effective (it's about 99.9%). It is reported that the vas deferens may recanalise spontaneously at a later time and result in an unexpected pregnancy in 1 : 2000.

Notes

If during surgery you fail to clearly identify the vas deferens on one side, it may not be necessarily your fault as there is a rare condition of **unilateral agenesis** of the vas deferens. In these circumstances it may be worth waiting for 16 weeks to check the sperm count before you proceed to scrotal exploration under general anaesthetic. If agenesis is indeed confirmed, arrange for an ultrasound scan of the kidneys, as this condition is also associated with **ipsilateral kidney agenesis**.

This is just one of the available vasectomy techniques. An alternative is the **scalpel-free** technique where a special sharp pointed instrument is used to make a single puncture in the median raphe from where the vas deferens from either side is delivered and ligated as explained. The term 'scalpel free' may be appealing to patients, but there is no difference in pain levels, and the cosmetic result is the same as small scars in the scrotum become invisible once healed.

For those men who change their mind at a later stage, either because of a loss of a child or spouse or any other change in their circumstances, there is an option of

reversal of vasectomy. This is most commonly seen in men under 30. Reversal of vasectomy is usually performed under general anaesthetic by specialised surgeons. The results are variable and **success rates drop significantly** the more time elapses from the original operation. It should therefore be made clear to men during the original consultation that, despite this option, vasectomy should be considered an irreversible procedure.

Summary

- With the patient **supine** and legs slightly **apart, examine** the genitals
- Inject a **nerve block**
- **Shave, prep** and **drape**
- **Hold the vas** and inject **local** into the overlying skin
- **Incise** the skin
- **Deliver** the vas deferens
- **Dissect** out a length of vas deferens
- **Clip** and **divide** the vas
- **Ligate** both ends, the proximal end **folded back**
- Ensure **haemostasis**
- **Close** the skin
- **Repeat** on the other side

20 Circumcision

Matt Stephenson and Matthew Fletcher

> **Video** | **12 min 6 s**
> Matthew Fletcher, Consultant Urologist
> Royal Sussex County Hospital, Brighton

Introduction

Considering the World Heath Organisation estimates that 30% of males worldwide are circumcised, circumcision must be up there as one of the most commonly performed operations in the world, and also one of the oldest. There are as many ways to do a circumcision as there are urologists, or so it's said. The way we demonstrate here is simple, gives an excellent cosmetic result and can be used on adults and children. Others have their own pet ways which they will vehemently defend. Learn one way of doing it and do it well.

Avoiding the wider debate regarding the indications for circumcision, the principal medical indications are **phimosis** and **paraphimosis**, for the former, particularly if you need access to the urethra for instance to do a cystoscopy or to catheterise.

Procedure

Prep the penis and the surrounding area with povidone iodine solution, under the foreskin too if it's retractable. **Drape** just the penis up to the base. Even if the patient is under general anaesthetic, a **penile block** will be appreciated by the patient postoperatively.

So to do the **penile block**, inject some 1% plain lignocaine (**never use adrenaline** in an appendage like the penis or finger with end arterial supply!) into the skin of the base of the penis in the midline and firstly just inject some local into the skin and **subcutaneous tissues**. Then **go deeper**, trying to catch the **dorsal nerves** of the penis as they run under the **pubic symphysis**, with 0.5% plain bupivocaine, the dose dependent on the patient's weight. But be careful, **aspirate first** to check you've not gone too deep and entered the **corpora cavernosa**. Once you've finished in the midline, **slide** the needle around each side of the base of the penis to catch the **ventral branches**. It infiltrates very easily without any resistance as long as you're in the right plane. Doing it like this, you can get a full penile

How to Operate: for MRCS Candidates and Surgical Trainees, First Edition. M. Stephenson. © 2011 John Wiley & Sons, Ltd.
Published 2011 by John Wiley & Sons, Ltd.

block from one single puncture site in the midline of the dorsum of the penis. Check it's worked before you start!

Now **mark** the skin. You want one circumferential line running around the penis, on the dorsal side, just proximal to the corona and as you come round the ventral side, let your mark pass distally towards the frenulum, thus making a V-shape.

Now take **three clips** and put these **at 2, 6 and 10 o'clock** onto the skin of the preputial orifice, which may be very stenosed if there is severe phimosis. Holding these out allows you to stretch the penis out. Now **incise** along the mark you've just made. Remember, penile skin is **very thin**, you only need to go just through skin, usually not so deep as to cut many vessels. Holding out clips at the 10 and 2 o'clock positions, cut with a pair of scissors along the **dorsal midline** from the preputial orifice up to your incision, joining up with it. The foreskin may be very **adherent** to the glans and may take a lot of persuasion to separate from it,

particularly if there has been longstanding balanitis. Take great care when performing this dorsal slit to ensure the jaws of the scissors **don't enter the urethral meatus**—that would be a disaster.

You can now **peel** the right and left sides of **the foreskin back**, a bit like peeling a banana, revealing the glans. If there was a tight phimosis before, you'll need to **clean the glans** with prep at this stage as clearly the field will no longer be sterile.

So remember the penile skin runs down from the shaft to the tip of the penis and then **rolls in on itself** to reinsert on the corona. The foreskin is therefore **double layered** over the glans. So far we've incised the outer layer just proximal to the corona, and now we've peeled the foreskin open we can access the inner layer of foreskin. So **put a clip** on to the edge of the peeled back foreskin on each side and hold up. You can now **incise the inner layer** of penile skin just **distal** to the corona leaving a good margin—and carry this all the way circumferentially round on each side to the frenulum.

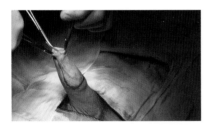

Three clips hold the prepuce up, note the line of incision has been marked. The line looks distal to the corona here only because the skin is being pulled up by the clips.

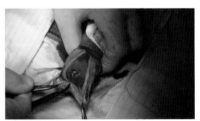

A dorsal slit has been made and the foreskin can peel back each side.

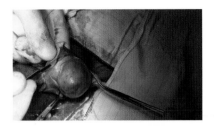

The inner layer of foreskin is being incised, leaving a good cuff of skin to stitch to later.

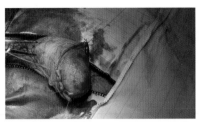

Note the stay stitches at 6 and 12 o'clock; a row of sutures is being inserted.

Both layers of foreskin have now been incised and the foreskin will just be flapping in the breeze, attached to the penis by a very thin layer of connective tissue between the outer and inner layers, which you can incise or snip with scissors, and also by a **stalk** to the frenulum. There's usually a vessel or two going up into the foreskin at the frenulum so it's best to **ligate** it here. Some people advocate a figure of eight suture here. Once this is divided, the foreskin is off—send it to histopathology.

Regarding **haemostasis**—it doesn't usually bleed too much as long as you don't cut too deeply as you're making your initial incision through the thin penile skin. Never use diathermy in children as there is a risk of thrombosing off the vessels in the corpora. If there are any bleeding vessels, make sure you deal with them, ideally by **ligating** them, before they retract back under the skin only to bleed in the recovery room.

So next, you need to **suture** the penile skin you initially incised circumferentially to that margin of inner foreskin you left around the corona. Begin on the **ventral side**, reattaching the **V-shaped flap** of skin up to the under-surface of the glans with one interrupted absorbable suture (like Vicryl Rapide), leave the end long and put a clip on it. Now get another suture at the **dorsal side**, that is at 12 o'clock— leave the end long and put a clip on it. Those clips at 6 and 12 o'clock serve as **stay stitches** to help control the penis so you can flop it to the left or right and allows you to do the next step: put a **line of interrupted sutures** on each side.

So then you just need to put a simple dressing on, firstly a **non-adhesive dressing** like Jelonet followed by **blue gauze** and tape. **Postoperatively**, advise them to **let the air get to it**, it doesn't matter if the dressing falls off on day 2, or in the car home which is more common. They should have **twice daily salt baths** and wear **loose clothing**; the sutures of course are **absorbable**. Make sure the patient has plenty of **analgesia** to take; it's sensible to start it **before** the block wears off.

Summary

- Whether under general anaesthetic or not, put in a **penile block**
- Mark a **circumferential line** just proximal to the corona moving into a V-shape over the frenulum
- Hold the preputial orifice with **clips** at 2, 6 and 10 o'clock
- **Incise** along the mark
- Make a **dorsal slit** with scissors and peel back the foreskin on each side
- Take a **clip** to each side
- Incise the **inner layer** of foreskin
- **Ligate** the vessels in the **frenulum**
- Send the foreskin to **histopathology**
- Put **stay sutures** at 6 (therefore reconstructing the frenulum) and 12 o'clock
- Insert a **row of interrupted sutures** down each side
- Put on a **non-adhesive dressing** and gauze

21 Nephrectomy

Matt Stephenson and Philip Thomas

> **Video** | **26 min 11 s**
> Philip Thomas, Consultant Urologist, supervising
> Shawket Alkhayal and Mamoun Elmoun
> Royal Sussex County Hospital, Brighton

Introduction

These days, like so many other surgical pathologies it seems the only nephrectomies that come to an open operation are the more difficult, complex ones. This is because **laparoscopic** approaches have gained so much in popularity. This is understandable given their quicker recovery times and reduced postoperative pain, but laparoscopic surgery is not always suitable for large, complex renal problems. This means of course that learning on an easy one is rather difficult for the trainee to do.

The commonest approach for a nephrectomy is through a **loin incision**. For very large kidneys or in cases of trauma, it may be easier to do through a **transabdominal approach** via either a midline laparotomy or transverse incision, which particularly allows early control of the vessels. If there's any preoperative concern that there may be extension of tumour into the inferior vena cava (IVC), it is usually safer to proceed with a **thoracoabdominal** incision so that access and control of the IVC above and below is possible.

Always remember, before embarking on removing someone's kidney, to make sure you've checked the overall renal function with **creatinine** levels and analysis of the **contralateral kidney** on imaging. If this is their only kidney you're taking out, or the other has poor function, you'll need to prepare for this with the support of the renal physicians.

Procedure

Before doing anything with the patient, fastidiously check you've got the **correct side**. Examine the patient, check the preoperatively made mark indicating the side, check the notes, check the consent form and check the imaging. This will be covered by the WHO surgical checklist (see *Patient Safety* Chapter 43), but you cannot be too careful.

The patient is under **general anaesthetic** with an **epidural catheter** and

How to Operate: for MRCS Candidates and Surgical Trainees, First Edition. M. Stephenson. © 2011 John Wiley & Sons, Ltd.
Published 2011 by John Wiley & Sons, Ltd.

urinary catheter *in situ*. She is **turned on her side** with the appropriate lumbar and arm supports with cushioning of all **pressure points** and tape to secure a **stable position**. The table needs to be **broken in the middle**, which means that both the head and feet are pointing down, which has the effect of stretching out the loin uppermost.

In deciding where to make the incision, it's best to **mark this out** with a pen first before prepping. **Palpate the 12th rib** and mark an outline of this. The incision needs to extend from the **superior surface** of the 12th rib and head **anteroinferiorly** in roughly the same line as the rib until beyond the anterior axillary line.

Prep and **drape** the loin. Make a final mental check that you're operating on the **correct kidney**. **Incise skin** through the previously made mark. Incise through **superficial fat** and go down onto the fascial covering of **external oblique**. Remember, laterally, the external oblique is an obvious muscle, unlike more anteriorly, such as in an appendicectomy, where you come across the aponeurotic

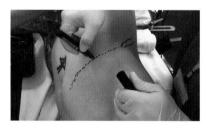

The patient is lying on her side facing to the left. The 12th rib is outlined posteriorly and the incision is extended anteromedially.

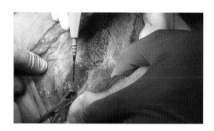

The artery forceps have been inserted beneath external oblique in preparation for division of the muscle (viewing from head end).

part. Locate the **tip of the 12th rib** and using the blunt ends of an artery forceps **puncture carefully** through the abdominal wall musculature on the superior side of the 12th rib. This will allow you an entry point to pass your artery forceps underneath the external oblique, lift it up and diathermy it on the stretch. **Divide** it with finger switch **diathermy**, stopping any bleeding points before they retract into the muscle belly. Repeat the process for the **internal oblique**, again making an entry point at the superior edge of the tip of the 12th rib—you can just put your fingers underneath it, or an artery forceps, to again lift it up and divide it on the stretch.

Why the superior part of the 12th rib? Because the **subcostal nerve** will run from inferior to the 12th rib. You want to avoid damaging it as the patient can develop an ugly swelling (which can look a bit like a hernia, but isn't) of the upper outer quadrant due to muscle laxity from this denervation. It runs between the internal oblique and transversus abdominus, so locate it in this plane and retract it inferolaterally out of the way.

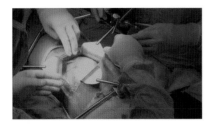

The Omnitract has been inserted, to do most of the work of retraction.

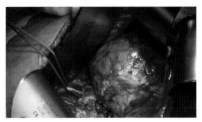

The blue vascular sloop has been slung around the ureter. The very large appearance of the kidney is due to a huge cyst which in this case needed to be drained to gain access to the hilum.

The final layer to open is the **transversus abdominus** muscle which can be split in the line of its fibres rather than cut. Next you'll come across **peritoneum**. Ordinarily, you'd probably be used to opening this layer to get to whatever pathology you wanted to access, but the kidneys of course are retroperitoneal. You need to **dissect into the retroperitoneal space** by retracting the **peritoneum anteromedially**. You should be able to find the most lateral part of the peritoneal reflection and peel it forwards revealing the kidney, covered by the yellow **Gerota's fat**. It doesn't really matter if you inadvertently perforate the peritoneum, you can repair any holes later, but do bear in mind how close colon can be. Usually at this stage, a large self-retaining retractor such as an **Omnitract** is very helpful and will make you popular with your assistants.

The first, safest place to start is usually to dissect around the **lower pole** looking out for two key structures: the **ureter** and the **gonadal vein**. Hunt around for these carefully, remembering that they can be pulled anteromedially with the peritoneum

you've been peeling off. Once you've found them, use Lahey forceps to get a **vascular sloop** around each of them. **Don't divide them yet**. If you find that this kidney is going to be irresectable, you'll need the ureter to continue draining it of urine. You can then **follow them up** superiorly by careful dissection. The ureter will take you to the hilum. On the left, the gonadal vein takes you to the left renal vein, on the right it takes you to the IVC. As you follow them, peel the **peritoneum off medially** until you reach the hilum. You'll be able to identify the **pancreas** and the **colon** being peeled out of the way. Once you've identified the **renal vein**, get a **vascular sloop round this** too. **Don't ligate it yet**, otherwise the renal artery will continue to pump blood into the kidney, with one less major exit resulting in congestion and potentially disastrous bleeding.

The next thing to do is get control of the renal artery, which lies **behind** the renal vein. Trying to identify it from the front, as you have for the vein, is tricky and potentially dangerous as it can be difficult to distinguish from the superior mesenteric artery. So now change tack and start to **dissect around the back** of the kidney, peeling the kidney anteromedially, looking for the **renal artery**, on the other side of the hilum. Once you've found it you need to meticulously check that it is indeed the renal artery and as such is definitely going into the renal substance and nowhere else. Imagine the consequences of misidentifying the superior mesenteric or even coeliac artery and dividing one of those. Once you're happy you've found it, **ligate it** with three strong (e.g. 0 Vicryl) ties leaving two on the aortic side and one on the kidney side. **Tie them well**, and leave a reasonable stump; a slipped ligature so close to the aorta would be catastrophic. **Repeat** the same process for the renal vein that you already slung a sloop round. If there are any other tributary veins such as the adrenal or a lumbar, tie or clip these too. Once you've assessed that the kidney is going to be resectable, you can **ligate**

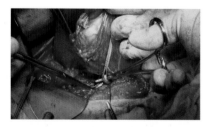

The renal artery has been slung with a blue sloop and is being ligated three times. Note the kidney has been reflected anteriorly (the camera angle here has returned to side on).

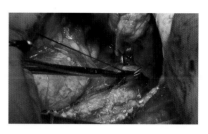

The Lahey forceps are around the renal vein in order to ligate it. The kidney is being retracted out to the right of the picture.

and divide the ureter and the **gonadal vein**.

The only part that remains to be dissected free is the **superior pole**. It's generally best to leave this until last because it can be close to the spleen, which can be an unforgiving organ even in seemingly minor iatrogenic trauma, so it's safer to do under **direct vision**, which you now can do with everything else freed up. As you're doing this, on the superior pole of the kidney you'll find a yellow blob of tissue—the **adrenal gland**. Either dissect this with your specimen if you're planning to take this too, or leave it behind (see the Notes section) dissecting in a plane between kidney and adrenal gland. **Divide any remaining strands** of tissue and send the kidney to the histopathologists. **Meticulously check** the kidney bed for **bleeding**, including the security of the ligatures on the tied ends of the vessels. If things seem a little oozy, with no actual bleeding point, consider leaving a **drain** in.

Remove the retractor, **unbreak the table** and **close up**. Close the abdominal wall muscles in **two layers**, firstly the

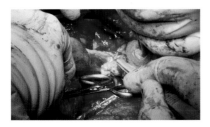

The left hand is retracting the kidney inferiorly whilst the diathermy forceps are on the yellow adrenal gland pulling it superiorly.

transversus and internal oblique together and secondly the **external oblique**, both with, for example PDS. The **skin** can then be closed with a continuous absorbable subcuticular stitch.

Notes

In cases where you suspect malignancy may have involved the **adrenal gland** by direct extension, the adrenal should be taken with the kidney. This would generally include upper pole or just large tumours or where there are abnormalities identified on imaging or intraoperatively.

Sometimes **tumour thrombus** (which is a mixture of tumour and thrombus) is found in the renal vein and you should be careful to dissect along the renal vein as far proximally as necessary to ensure you ligate it beyond such thrombus. This occasionally means as far as into the **IVC**.

Summary

- Check the **correct side**
- **Position** the patient comfortably on their side with the **table broken**
- **Mark** the incision
- **Prep** and **drape**
- **Re-check** the side
- Make the **skin incision**
- **Deepen** through **fat**
- Make an **entry point** at the tip of the **12th rib**
- Divide **external oblique**, then **internal oblique**
- Identify and protect the **subcostal nerve**
- Split **transversus abdominus**
- Insert **Omnitract**
- **Reflect peritoneum** anteromedially
- Dissect **inferior pole**
- Identify and sling **ureter** and **gonadal vein**
- **Trace up** to **hilum**
- Identify and sling **renal vein**
- Dissect round **back of kidney** to find **renal artery**
- **Sling renal artery** and confirm its identity
- **Ligate renal artery** x 3 and divide
- **Ligate renal vein** x 3 and divide
- Dissect around **superior pole**
- Remove or preserve **adrenal gland**
- Send kidney to **histopathology**
- Check for **haemostasis** and consider **drain**
- Close **internal oblique** and **transversus** together
- Close **external oblique**
- Close **skin**

22 Dynamic Hip Screw

Matt Stephenson and Lisa Leonard

> **Video** | **8 min 49 s**
> Lisa Leonard, Consultant Orthopaedic Surgeon,
> supervising R. Vaidyalinga Sharma
> Royal Sussex County Hospital, Brighton

Introduction

For a discussion about hip fractures in general see *Hemiarthroplasty* Chapter 23. So when should you perform a **dynamic hip screw (DHS)** and when should you perform a **hemiarthroplasty** for a **fractured neck of femur**? The choice depends on whether or not the fracture is likely to compromise the blood supply to the femoral head resulting in **avascular necrosis**. Remember that the **blood supply** to the femoral head comes from three principle sources: (1) through the **foveolar artery** in the ligamentum teres (not usually affected by a hip fracture and doesn't supply much blood anyway so clinically irrelevant, except in children); (2) the **nutrient artery** of the shaft; and (3) the **retinacular vessels** that run within the hip joint capsule, these are the most important ones.

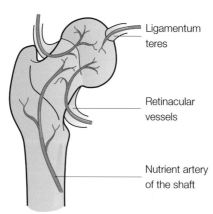

Ligamentum teres

Retinacular vessels

Nutrient artery of the shaft

The blood supply of the femoral head.

How to Operate: for MRCS Candidates and Surgical Trainees, First Edition. M. Stephenson. © 2011 John Wiley & Sons, Ltd. Published 2011 by John Wiley & Sons, Ltd.

Types of hip fracture

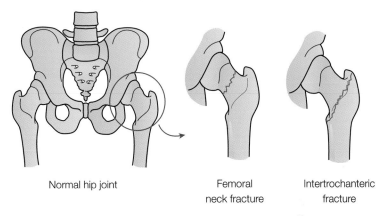

Normal hip joint   Femoral   Intertrochanteric
neck fracture   fracture

Types of hip fracture—extracapsular and intracapsular.

Femoral neck fractures can be broadly divided into **intracapsular** and **extra-capsular**. Remember that the capsule inserts **low down** on the femoral neck, perhaps lower than you might think (as can be seen in the figure). **Intracapsular** fractures are then classified by the **Garden classification** into four stages.

In **Garden 1 and 2**, the femoral head should still be perfused by a combination principally of the retinacular vessels and to a lesser extent the nutrient artery. Therefore all that is required is to fix the fracture site to give it time to heal—a **dynamic hip screw** is indicated. If the head is displaced however, that is **Garden 3 and 4**, then the nutrient artery will certainly have been torn, as almost certainly will the retinacular vessels as the capsule will also have been torn. The femoral head, even if you fix it in place, will die. Replacement of the femoral head is indicated—a **hemiarthroplasty**. You can use the

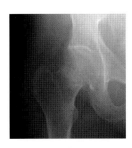 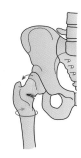

Stage 1: A valgus impacted fracture, and undisplaced.

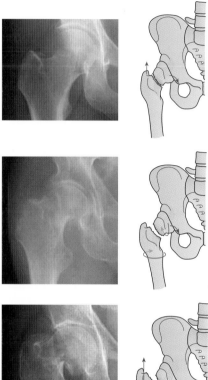

Stage 2: Complete fracture of the neck but undisplaced.

Stage 3: Complete fracture and partially displaced, because the femoral head is still hinged onto the shaft to some extent, the bony trabeculae of the femoral head no longer line up with those of the adjacent acetabulum.

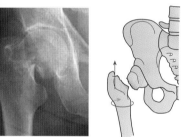

Stage 4: Complete fracture and completely displaced, now the head is free to rotate back to the anatomical position in the acetabulum and the trabeculae lines now line up again.

The Garden classification of intracapsular fractures.

mnemonic: **one, two: screw; three, four: Austin–Moore**. This is a slight over simplification, see the Notes section.

In **extracapsular fractures**, the retinacular vessels will still be intact and all that is required is fixation of the fracture, hence a **dynamic hip screw** is needed in these patients.

Procedure

The patient is under either **general** or **spinal anaesthetic** and **supine** on an orthopaedic traction table. The **feet** are **secured in stirrups** allowing the legs to be manipulated into various positions.

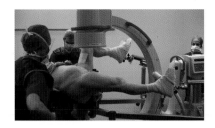

The patient is on an orthopaedic traction table with the affected leg on traction, abduction and internally rotated. The unaffected leg is abducted allowing the II to easily view the hip. Note the traction groin post between the patients legs, this allows traction to be applied to the leg without the patient falling off the table—take care of the genitals though.

There are numerous joints and adaptable components on this equipment making it very versatile. The first thing to do in a displaced fracture is to **reduce the fracture;** obviously you don't want to fix it into an abnormal position. To do this, put **traction** on the affected leg and apply **internal rotation** to it so that the patella is facing the ceiling.

Clearly you're going to need to have X-ray vision to see whether you've returned it to a satisfactory position. And that's what the **image intensifier** (affectionately known as the **II**) is there for. It is shaped like a large C, emitting X rays from one end with an X-ray detector on the other end. By abducting the unaffected leg widely, you can get the II into position to view the fracture site in both **anteroposterior** (AP) and **lateral** views. Make sure that there's nothing obstructing the movement of the II so that it can be

easily changed to the AP or lateral positions during the course of the operation. Of course, if the fracture is undisplaced, you can fix it where it is without any manipulation.

Once you're happy with the position, **prep** the whole of the thigh and surrounding areas and apply a **drape** to the upper lateral thigh. This drape is pretty huge with a sticky bit for the operative site and peripherally to this is a large transparent plastic sheet which can be fixed to some drip stands and an intervening horizontal bar or similar equipment in order to give a very large sterile wall from floor to above standing height. It also has a collecting pouch beneath the operative field that will help to collect any blood dripping out of the wound, stopping it getting to the floor.

So now make the **skin incision;** this should be about 15 cm long commencing just behind the palpable **greater trochanter** continuing **longitudinally** down the thigh over the lateral femur (often easily palpable in thin old ladies). Cut

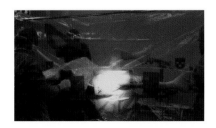

The operative site is draped with a large sterile drape attached to drip stands and an overhead bar.

straight down through **subcutaneous fat**, maintaining haemostasis as you go. The first obvious layer you see will be the **fascia lata**—an obvious white fascial layer. Incise straight through this. Inserting a **self-retaining retractor** such as a Travers or in a deeper wound, a Norfolk and Norwich retractor (or even two) will help exposure.

The next layer is the **vastus lateralis**. This can be retracted anteriorly and approached from behind but this can result in lots of bleeding because of an abundance of perforating vessels posteriorly, so simply **split it** in line with its fibres. First, **cut the fascial envelope** of the muscle with a knife and then **bluntly dissect** your way through the muscle. Replace the self-retaining retractor within the muscle and you will find yourself down onto the **periosteum**-covered **lateral femur**. There will be strands of muscle attached to the surface too, so **strip** all these off with a periosteal elevator, including the periosteum, to give a broad surface of upper lateral femur to later place the plate of the DHS device on to.

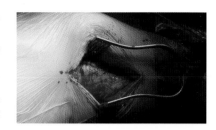

Fascial covering of vastus lateralis is exposed.

Apply an **angle guide** to the lateral femur and feel the anterior and posterior edges and make sure you're in the middle. Insert the guide pin through the appropriate hole which will give you a 135 degree angle into the femoral neck, matching that on your plate. Once your guide and pin are laid against the bone, take an X ray to check the position.

Drill the guide pin into the femur a few centimetres, keeping the angle guide firmly pressed against the femoral shaft and directing it just very slightly anteriorly, as the head is usually slightly anteverted on the shaft (you can see this on the lateral

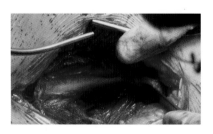

A periosteal elevator has scraped off the muscle to expose the lateral surface of femur.

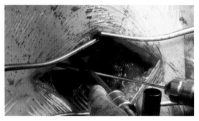

Angle guide is placed over the lateral surface of the femur. The guide pin is seen passing obliquely on to the femoral surface.

film). **Take another X ray** in the AP position and check that it's advancing in the right direction. If it is, keep drilling it into the femur with regular X rays to check its position. You're aiming for dead centre within the femoral head. If it's going in the wrong direction, reposition the angle guide, checking its flat against the femoral shaft. Once you've gone some way in towards the femoral neck, **re-position the II** to check the **lateral view**. Sometimes you think you're doing a great job and the angle looks great in the AP view, and then change to the lateral and realise you've gone out the back of the hip altogether. So the guide pin must be going directly up the axis of the femoral neck in both views. If not, correct it early by withdrawing, repositioning and re-drilling. Get the tip of the guide pin up to the **subchondral surface** of the femoral head. The crucial distance to estimate is the 'tip–apex' distance. This is the distance from the pin to the centre of the femoral head surface. Add this measurement from both the AP and lateral views

and the total should come to less than 25 mm. This reduces the chance of the screw cutting out.

Once you're happy with the position in both views you may wish to insert an antirotation guide pin. The purpose of this is to prevent the femoral head from spinning around when you come to the next step, reaming. **Remove the angle guide**.

Once you've got a guide pin in the right position, you need to **measure the length** of screw you need. Slide a **measuring device** over the exposed guide pin down to where it vanishes inside the femur. This is specially calibrated to give a length of screw needed by determining how much guide pin is inside by subtracting how much is left outside. Ask for the screw at this stage at the same length as your measurement but ask for the reamer to be set at 5–10 mm less than the measurement. Check the reamer length you are given and feed it over the guide pin and **ream out** the space for the screw to go in, checking on the II that

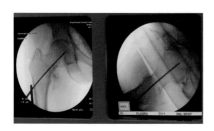

On the left, the AP view is seen and on the right the lateral view, with the guide pin in an acceptable position.

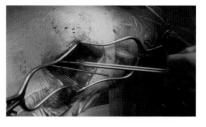

You can see two guide pins here, the second is to stop the femoral head from spinning when the screw is screwed in. The measuring device is being fed over the primary guide pin.

Dynamic Hip Screw | **117**

the pin hasn't been pushed in through the acetabulum.

Now **insert the screw** into the reamed-out space and **screw it in firmly** so that the screw engages deep within the femoral head. Once it's in position, the handle of the screwing device should be **parallel** with the axis of the femur. This is important because the end of the screw is shaped to engage with the plate in this orientation, thus preventing rotation of the femoral head once the plate is in place. **Confirm the position** throughout with the II.

Next **slide the barrel** of the **plate** down over the distal end of the screw and

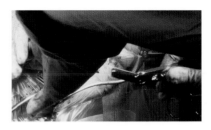

The barrel of the plate is about to be threaded over the screw.

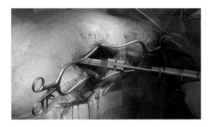

The reamer is threaded over the primary guide pin.

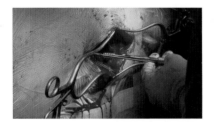

The dynamic hip screw is threaded over the guide pin and screwed into place.

lay it down along the long axis of the femur, make sure there are no strands of muscle interposed between it and the femur. Because of the shape of the screw, the plate will fit onto it and not be able to rotate, however, the screw will be able to **slide in and out** of the buttress plate, hence the term dynamic, and this allows the fracture site to **collapse**, **compress** together and **unite**. Using an orthopaedic **mallet**, hammer the buttress plate firmly into position.

There are several holes along the plate to accommodate the screws. Check that the most distal screw hole lines up with the femur. The first thing to do is **drill a hole** all the way through the femur through the proximal plate hole. You'll feel the resistance in drilling whilst going through the **lateral cortex** and then a give as it passes through this as the drill passes easily through the soft **medullary canal**. There will then be another wall of resistance as it engages the **medial cortex**—drill through this and there will be another give of overcoming resistance as you pass through the other side of the

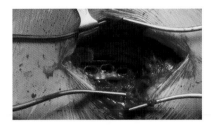

The plate lying against the femur—the holes are about to accommodate screws.

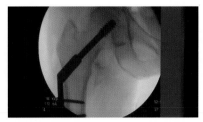

Final position of dynamic hip screw. A further image should be taken inferiorly to check the position of the other screws.

femur—so obviously stop as soon as you feel this. Remove the drill and insert a **depth gauge**. This consists of a long central pin with a hooked end that you pass straight through your drill hole out the other side of the femur and then pull back allowing the hook to get caught on the outer surface of the medial cortex. There is then an outer component that slides down over the central pin to abut the surface of the buttress plate allowing you to measure the depth the pin has gone in and thus the length of screw required.

Repeat this for all the screw holes and **screw** the appropriately sized screws into position. **Check the final position** of the dynamic hip screw, buttress plate and femoral screws with the II.

Irrigate the wound with normal saline to remove any fragments of bone that can act as a nidus for infection and check for **haemostasis**. **Close the fascial** **envelope** of the vastus lateralis and then the **fascia lata** with absorbable sutures. Closing the fat layer is optional but then **close the skin** with a subcuticular absorbable continuous suture.

Notes

In young and fit patients (for example under 40) a displaced subcapital fracture is an emergency, and you want to try and retain the femoral head if at all possible. This may mean accepting the higher risk of avascular necrosis with cannulated screws or a short dynamic hip screw with an antirotation screw. In a slightly older age group, but still fit, a total hip replacement might be a better option as these give better long-term functional results. Uncemented hemiarthroplasties are now usually reserved for medically unfit, poorly mobile patients. Cemented hemiarthroplasty or bipolar prostheses are other options.

Summary

- The patient is under **general anaesthetic** or **spinal, supine** on an **orthopaedic traction table**
- **Reduce the fracture** and abduct the unaffected leg
- **Position the II** and **confirm reduced position** in AP and lateral views
- Make **skin incision**
- **Incise** through **fat**, **fascia lata** and **vastus lateralis**
- **Scrape muscle** and **periosteum** off femur
- **Drill guide pin** using **angle guide**
- **Confirm position** with II in both dimensions
- Consider **inserting second pin** if risk of femoral head rotation
- **Measure size** of screw
- **Ream** appropriate size space for screw
- **Screw in dynamic hip screw**
- **Confirm position** with II
- Insert **buttress plate**
- **Drill holes** in femoral shaft and **measure depth**
- **Screw** in appropriately sized screws
- **Check position**
- **Irrigate** and **close in layers**

23 Hip Hemiarthroplasty

Matt Stephenson and Lisa Leonard

> **Video** | **16 min 50 s**
> Lisa Leonard, Consultant Orthopaedic Surgeon,
> supervising R. Vaidyalinga Sharma
> Royal Sussex County Hospital, Brighton

Introduction

Few operations are performed on more elderly or frail patients than in the case of fixing a fractured neck of femur. When you consider that the 6-month survival following a hip fracture is in the region of **70%**, it gives you an idea of the kind of protoplasm you're dealing with. It's not the hip fracture itself that kills the patient—it will be one of the complications of the resulting diminution of mobility, whatever caused the fall in the first place or other co-morbidities.

There is a lot you can do to improve the lot of this elderly cohort of patients—and it's not just about doing a good operation with technical success in a timely manner. These often vulnerable patients need optimal medical therapy, in terms of resuscitation after hours spent on the floor, antibiotics for their urine infection or cardiological assessment for their dysrhythmias.

There are two principle approaches to the hip: **anterolateral (Hardinge approach)**, which is discussed and shown here, or the **posterior approach**, which utilises an incision slightly more posteriorly and instead of going through the abductors, you cut through the external rotators of the hip. It has the purported benefit of less damage to the abductors, which tends to result in a Trendelenburg gait, but can have a higher risk of injury to the sciatic nerve. Very few people would use this approach for a hemiarthroplasty, it is more used for a total hip replacement.

Procedure

The patient is under **general anaesthetic** or **spinal** in the **lateral position** with the fractured hip uppermost. Careful **positioning** is very important to ensure stability (i.e. the reaming or hammering isn't going to end up with the patient on the floor), that **pressure points** are protected and that the pelvis is clearly oriented on the table. **Thromboembolic**

How to Operate: for MRCS Candidates and Surgical Trainees, First Edition. M. Stephenson. © 2011 John Wiley & Sons, Ltd.
Published 2011 by John Wiley & Sons, Ltd.

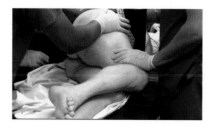

The right lateral position for a fractured right neck of femur. Note the urinary catheter *in situ*.

prophylaxis is particularly important given the high rates of deep vein thrombosis (DVT) post hip surgery so pneumatic compression stockings on the contralateral leg is sensible if not contraindicated. Most people recommend a urinary catheter is placed intraoperatively if not already inserted as it will be very painful to use a bedpan or commode, and also helps monitor urinary output in these usually elderly, frail patients.

Infection of any prosthesis in general is a disaster. Infection of a prosthetic hip is no exception—it is an unmitigated disaster which may result in the prosthesis having to come out, washouts, long-term antibiotics, considerable morbidity or death. Attention to **sterility** is therefore paramount. If you accidentally desterilise yourself on your way from the sink to the operating table on your first day with your new boss—own up to it and rescrub. **Clean the skin** widely with a soapy solution just to reduce the infective load, dry it and then re-prep formally once you've scrubbed.

A **U-shaped drape** is useful to wrap around the upper thigh, exposing the hip and drape the foot separately and bandage it—you'll need to move that leg around later on with some special manoeuvres. Stand on the side with the patient facing away from you. Many people also cover the skin with an **adhesive translucent drape** (e.g. Ioban), which can be incised through and reduces the number of skin commensals that can be knocked off into the wound.

Before you make your incision through skin, **identify some bony landmarks**. Palpate the **greater trochanter**—the most prominent bony bit of the hip. Inferior to that palpate the **shaft of the femur** descending down the thigh. You want your incision to extend from the greater trochanter **straight down inferiorly** over the middle of the shaft and superiorly from the greater trochanter **curving slightly posteriorly** (rather than continuing in a straight line as this will give better access

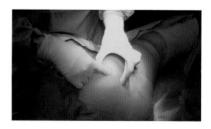

The assistant's right hand is pointing to the greater trochanter whilst the left hand is palpating the shaft of the femur.

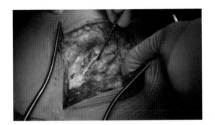

The fascia lata is being incised.

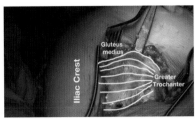

The gluteus medius has been labelled along with its attachments to the iliac crest and the greater trochanter. A McDonald dissector has been inserted underneath this muscle, which on this individual is very thin.

to the acetabulum). **Incise** through **skin** and **subcutaneous fat** down to **fascia lata** (the deep fascia of the thigh). Cut straight through that to find the **tensor fascia lata** (a strip of muscle attached superiorly to the iliac crest inserting onto the fascia lata) and cut through this.

The next layer you'll face is the **abductors** of the hip—the **gluteus medius** and **minimus**—descending from the iliac crest above down and slightly posteriorly to the greater trochanter of the hip. Firstly you'll cut through gluteus medius and deep to it, although you may not be able to separately identify it, will be the gluteus minimus. Divide gluteus medius by keeping one-third of it inferoposteriorly and the remaining two-thirds superoanteriorly. As usual when dividing muscles—they have a tendency to bleed—so use **diathermy**.

As you're dividing through it, ask your assistant to apply external rotation to the thigh and as the final fibres are cut, the upper part of the femur will then flop out laterally **exposing the fractured neck** of the femur, which may be covered by some **hip capsule** which you can divide. You can then turn the thigh into external

rotation and adduction and the foot can be allowed to hang over the other side of the bed with the tibia hanging vertically into the pouch in the drape—which pulls out the upper femur into the wound.

In order to fit the prosthesis in, you'll need to remove the part of the femur roughly above the **intertrochanteric line**. Take an implant and lay it over the upper part of the femur roughly where it is going to lie and **mark the periosteum** with diathermy. This will be the line running along where the flange of the implant will run, which will be roughly from greater

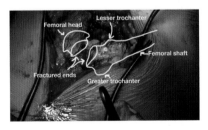

The view as you look into the wound with an overlay of where the bones lay.

trochanter to lesser trochanter. Take an **electric saw** and cut off everything above this line, except the most lateral bit where the greater trochanter is (to preserve some of the attachments of the abductors). With that out of the way, peer into the depths of the wound and you'll be able to see the fractured surface of the neck attached to the femoral head, deep in the acetabulum. Insert a **corkscrew femoral head extractor** into the middle of the fracture surface and screw it in deeply and **pluck out** the femoral head (it's attached to the acetabulum only by the ligamentum teres).

Measure the extracted femoral head to **size the new implant**—an **Austin–Moore** is shown in the video, an **uncemented** prosthesis (a Thompson hemiarthroplasty is an example of a cemented option, for which the neck is also slightly different). The size of the head and the shaft can be selected. The shaft can be in standard or narrow widths—the vast majority take a standard. Whilst your chosen size prosthesis is being found, **ream** the femoral shaft.

Use a **box chisel** to fashion the trochanter to fit the implant. Reaming involves inserting a special instrument called a **rasp** with edges that shave off the bone as it is hammered down the inside of the femoral shaft. The idea is that it creates a space in the femoral shaft that will allow the implant to fit exactly. **Wash out** any fragments of bone—how would you like loose chips of bone and debris in your acetabulum?

Take your **implant** and **insert** it down the femoral shaft—it should now fit snugly but may need to be **hammered** home with an **impacter** to protect the prosthetic head. Now to **relocate** the new hip. Up until now the hip has been grossly adducted and externally rotated. Reduce it by taking the foot out of the pouch applying longitudinal traction and slowly internally rotating the head back in to the acetabulum—take care at this stage, forcible rotation can break the femur—you'll hear it **clunking** into the acetabulum. **Check the leg lengths** by comparing the positions of the knees. Now test the **stability** of the hip by moving it

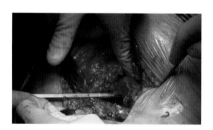 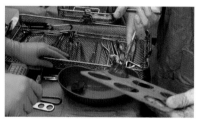

The cork screw has been driven into the femoral head (the camera angle has changed, you're now looking from the foot end), has plucked it out and then checked for size using a head sizer.

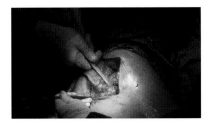

The reamer has been inserted down the femoral shaft.

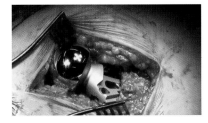

The implant is inserted down the femoral shaft.

into the various positions—most crucially full **internal rotation** and **external rotation** whilst the hip is adducted.

Now to **close the layers**, but first **irrigate** the wound again with some saline to remove any remaining debris and reduce the risk of infection. Put a stitch or two in the **hip capsule** itself; this should reduce the risk of dislocation. **Close the abductors** with an absorbable suture and then another continuous layer to the **fascia lata**. If there is a significant **fat layer**, close it with another layer of continuous absorbable suture with a final subcuticular layer for **skin** and **Steristrips**.

Summary

- The patient is under **general anaesthetic** or **spinal** in the **lateral position**
- **Prep** and **drape** to expose the hip and thigh
- Identify the **greater trochanter** and the **femoral shaft**
- Make a **curvilinear incision**
- Incise through **skin**, **fat**, **fascia lata** and **tensor fascia lata**
- Incise through the **hip abductors**
- **Manoeuvre** the leg to bring out the distal fracture site
- **Shape** the upper femur for the implant
- **Pluck out** the femoral head
- **Size the implant**
- **Ream** the femoral shaft
- **Washout**
- **Insert implant**
- **Relocate**
- Test **stability** and **length**
- **Close the layers**

24 Carpal Tunnel Decompression

Matt Stephenson and Anand P Joshi

> **Video** | **7 min 22 s**
> Anand P Joshi, Consultant Orthopaedic Surgeon
> Medway Maritime Hospital, Gillingham

Introduction

Carpal tunnel syndrome is a very common condition—there are therefore plenty of opportunities to get your hands on one, usually as part of either an orthopaedic or neurosurgical job. It is a simple procedure and long considered a good way of cutting your teeth in day-case surgery.

To sum up the problem of carpal tunnel syndrome—the median nerve is squashed within the fixed space of the carpal tunnel. There is a long list of aetiologies, all with the common pathway of raising pressure within the carpal tunnel and this affects the microcirculation of the median nerve disturbing axonal transport with resultant pain, paraesthesia and weakness. The cure is simple—divide the one dividable structure of the osteofascial ring surrounding the carpal tunnel, the **flexor retinaculum**.

Procedure

The patient is **awake** with her arm laid out **fully supinated** on an arm board with the fingers outstretched. A **proximal tourniquet** is applied to the upper arm to keep the wound dry during the procedure. **Prep** and **drape** the hand and forearm.

Identify the **distal wrist crease** (there's also a proximal and middle one, in case you were interested). Next identify **Kaplan's** cardinal line—what on earth is that? Place the hand in the anatomical position with the **thumb extended and abducted**, pointing away from the palm. Imagine a **straight line** running from the ulnar border of the thumb across the palm to the hook of the hamate—this is Kaplan's line. The incision needs to run from a couple of millimetres distal to the distal wrist crease to Kaplan's line, and it should be in line with the third web space,

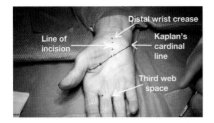

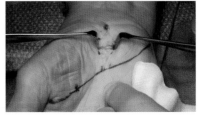

The relevant skin markings.

Retraction of subcutaneous fat.

that is the radial border of the ring finger or the ulnar border of the middle finger.

Inject local anaesthetic along this line (or this can be done before prepping to give it more time to work, as in the video) and **incise** through **skin** and **subcutaneous fat** and you'll soon come down to the **palmar aponeurosis**, with its fibres running in the **same direction** as your wound. **Incise them** in the line of the wound. Inserting a small self-retaining retractor, such as a **West retractor**, will help. Deep to this you will find the **flexor retinaculum**—a **white fibrous band** running **transversely** across the wrist—note the fibres running at 90 degrees to your wound.

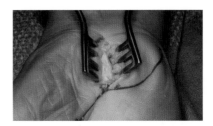

Exposure of palmar fascia.

Get a **McDonald dissector** underneath the flexor retinaculum to protect the underlying median nerve and **cut** straight down **through the flexor retinaculum** onto the McDonald dissector. Sometimes it's easiest to just make a small incision in the flexor retinaculum and then pass the McDonald dissector through the hole, proximally then distally. Feel the **crunchiness** of the flexor retinaculum as it's divided. One of the biggest reasons for failure of this procedure is inadequately dividing the retinaculum and this usually is at the proximal end of the incision—make sure there is no strand of fibrous tissue remaining here or at the distal end and that you can clearly see the underlying median nerve.

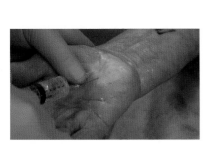

Injection of lignocaine with adrenaline (note the blanching of the skin).

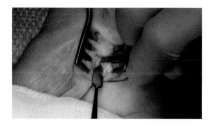

McDonald dissector inserted beneath the retinaculum, and the knife is cutting down onto it.

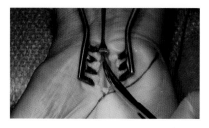

The proximal limit of the retinaculum is being inspected directly and divided.

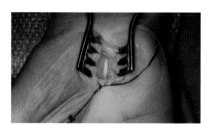

The freed median nerve.

Close only **the skin**, not the palmar aponeurosis. **Dress** the wound and wrap the wrist in a **wool** and **crepe** bandage; once the pressure is applied to the wound from the bandage, **release the tourniquet**.

Notes

There are **three important structures** to avoid damaging. **Proximally** the **cutaneous branch of the median nerve** is at risk. This is a branch of the median nerve that arises proximal to the flexor retinaculum and then runs superficially over it to supply the skin over the thenar eminence. Damage to it can result in a painful neuroma. The best way to avoid this is to not stray any further radial/ lateral during the incision or dissection. Its surface marking is roughly in line with the second web space. Also proximally is the **recurrent motor branch of the median nerve**—its course is variable but again providing you don't stray any further radial/ lateral, it should be safe.

Distally the structure at risk is the **superficial palmar arch**—the biggest of the two palmar arches. The apex of this arch runs roughly along Kaplan's line, therefore you need to be careful at the distal extent of the dissection.

Endoscopic carpal tunnel decompression is a newer technique and involves either a one- or two-incision procedure.

Summary

- The patient is **awake** with the arm **supinated** on an **armboard**
- **Prep** and **drape**
- Inject **local anaesthetic** in a line along the radial border of the index finger from just distal to the distal wrist crease to Kaplan's line
- **Incise** along the same line
- Incise through **subcutaneous fat** and **palmar aponeurosis**
- **Protect the median nerve** with the McDonald dissector
- **Divide** the **flexor retinaculum**
- Ensure **haemostasis**
- **Close skin**
- **Dress, bandage** and **release tourniquet**

25 Gastrectomy

Matt Stephenson and Peter C Hale

> **Video** | **30 min 27 s**
> Peter C Hale, Consultant General and Upper
> GI Surgeon
> Royal Sussex County Hospital, Brighton

Introduction

It's quite possible you've never been formally introduced to the stomach. You may have been around for a number of laparotomies and merely glimpsed it lurking up there under the ribs. You may have run a cursory hand over it when examining the abdominal contents or checking the position of the nasogastric tube. However, you are unlikely, unless you've been very lucky, to have had any more than a passing acquaintance with this interesting viscus.

It wasn't always like this, the stomach has felt long neglected by surgeons ever since the advent of medical therapy to control peptic ulcer disease. Peptic ulcers used to be dealt with surgically, either by prophylactic vagotomies or emergently when they perforated, and this is now comparatively rare. In the olden days, gastrectomies for large benign gastric ulceration were relatively common. Furthermore, the centralisation of upper gastrointestinal services has meant that gastrectomies for malignancy are happening in fewer centres.

So does all that mean you don't have to know how to take out the stomach? I'm afraid not, despite the relative rarity of gastrectomies now, every general surgeon needs to be able to do a gastrectomy in the emergency situation, mainly for those few remaining large, perforated gastric ulcers that are too big to simply be covered in an omental patch.

The only kind of gastrectomy you're likely to need if you're not an upper gastro-intestinal surgeon is a distal gastrectomy. You may have heard of the **Bilroth I** gastrectomy which involved doing a distal gastrectomy and then anastomosing the gastric remnant straight onto the duodenum but this has fallen out of favour. The **Bilroth II** or **Polya** gastrectomy, where the stomach is instead anastomosed onto nearby jejunum and the duodenum merely closed off, is what you need to know.

How to Operate: for MRCS Candidates and Surgical Trainees, First Edition. M. Stephenson. © 2011 John Wiley & Sons, Ltd.
Published 2011 by John Wiley & Sons, Ltd.

Procedure

With the patient **supine** under **general anaesthetic, shave, prep** and **drape** the whole of the abdomen. Make an **upper midline laparotomy**. Examine the abdominal contents, if you're doing this for known malignancy start by touching everything else in the abdomen rather than the cancer to reduce the risk of **seeding** it all over the peritoneum. In many centres, the patient will have had a **preoperative laparoscopy** to assess whether there is any evidence of spread before making a big hole in the abdomen.

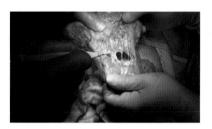

The omentum is being lifted superiorly and the transverse colon inferiorly; the lesser sac is then entered through the back of the omentum.

The general events in any gastrointestinal resection are to **mobilise** the viscus, **ligate and divide** its blood supply, **resect** it at the appropriate margins and **join two ends** together again. The gastrectomy is no different. The first step then is to begin mobilising the stomach and you do this by starting with the omentum.

Observe the **gastrocolic omentum** running down from the stomach to the transverse colon and then note the **greater omentum** (from herein just referred to as the omentum) hanging down from the transverse colon towards the pelvis. **Lift up the omentum** and pull it **superiorly,** exposing the back of the omentum as it meets the transverse colon. This is the place to begin. **Make a hole in the omentum** close to the transverse colon, this area is usually quite **avascular**. However, you need to remember that the omentum is not the only thing stuck onto the transverse colon—it has its own blood supply in the form of the **transverse mesocolon** which hangs down from the front of the pancreas. Often the omentum and mesocolon get **stuck together** and you only want to divide omentum without **devascularising** the transverse colon.

Once you've opened that omentum you've entered the **lesser sac**. You can't quite remember what that is can you? Consider you shrunk yourself down to the size of a pea and somehow slipped into the peritoneal cavity. You can roam around the peritoneal cavity to your heart's content, sliding down bowel loops and skipping up and down paracolic gutters, but it's quite unlikely that you would accidentally find yourself in the lesser sac unless you knew where to look. The lesser sac is a much smaller compartment of the peritoneal cavity hidden away behind the stomach. It is in continuity with the greater sac (where you've been playing) but only via a quite narrow entrance called the **foramen of Winslow**—the borders of which are: **anteriorly,** the free border of the lesser omentum; **posteriorly,** the inferior vena cava; **inferiorly,** the duodenum; and **superiorly,** the caudate lobe of the liver. Once you'd rolled yourself through that gateway you'd find yourself in a much cosier space, you might like to lie down for a while on the posterior wall in which case you would have the pancreas as a mattress with the transverse meso-colon hanging off the end of the bed. Directly facing you would be the back of the stomach and gastrocolic mesen-tery merging inferiorly with the omentum hanging off the transverse colon. If you looked to your left you would see the left kidney and adrenal gland. If you looked to the right you would see where you just came in. Just as you're dozing off, a giant firestick emerges towards you through the omentum forcing you to flee.

So, **open the lesser sac** widely now by dividing the omentum along the trans-verse colon, lift up the transverse colon and peer into the lesser sac. You should see the **back wall of the stomach** and the **salmon pink pancreas** directly behind this. Sometimes there are some **loose adhesions** between the two which you can divide, but this next step is crucial to assessing whether the stomach is resectable—can you put your hand between the two viscera? Note in the *Gastrojejunostomy* video we had to

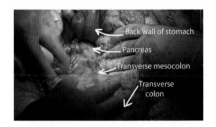

The stomach with attached omentum has been lifted upwards to reveal the back wall of the lesser sac.

abandon the gastrectomy at this stage, because the stomach cancer had invaded through into the pancreas, which makes it irresectable and the plan needs to change to a palliative procedure. Assum-ing you're happy to proceed with a resection, **complete the division** of the omentum off the colon on the right hand side, pushing the colon down and lifting the omentum up.

Now **identify the pylorus**. Often there is a white, slightly indented line running vertically, along with the **prepyloric vein of Mayo** and this marks the pylorus. You can **feel** between finger and thumb for a **circle of muscle** at this level. Once you've found this, the next step is to divide the tissue holding the pylorus and first part of the duodenum down **inferiorly;** in this tissue is the **right gastroepiploic artery**. There are also often a lot of other little vessels in this region which bleed if you're not careful. In the presence of a perforated ulcer in this region, clearly identifying the anatomy can be very difficult. **Ligate this leash** of tissue and you'll find you can lift the pylorus and first part of the duodenum superiorly.

Now turn your attention to the tissue coming in to the **superior** part of the duodenum and pylorus, the **lesser omentum**. In the free edge of this (more lateral than you would want to be) is the triad of portal vein, common hepatic duct and common hepatic artery—stay well clear of this. Instead **ligate and divide** the lesser omentum just above the pylorus and first part of the duodenum; here you will find the **right gastric artery**—a less juicy vessel than the right gastroepiploic. You'll now find you could curl your finger right round the first part of the duodenum, and this will allow you to insert a linear stapling device across the first part of the duodenum, just beyond the pylorus. You don't need to staple far beyond the pylorus even for cancer as it rarely spreads beyond the pylorus and, if it has, the resection is unlikely to be curative. So **staple across the first part of the duodenum**. Suddenly, you can lift up the stomach and its attached omentum incredibly freely.

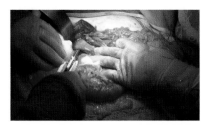

One limb of the stapling device has been placed round the back of the duodenum.

Pull down on it and decide how proximally you want to divide it. Generally speaking, you want to resect **one-half to two-thirds** of the stomach. The rationale for removing so much is that you reduce the chance of developing **stomal ulceration** because of excessive acid production. If you look at the arcade of vessels coming into the greater curvature of the stomach, you'll see the majority of them run from below and course **upwards** from the **left gastroepiploic artery**. There is a level some distance up the greater curvature, however, at which the gastroepiploic artery no longer feeds the stomach and the supply comes from the **short gastric arteries** which course from **superiorly to inferiorly**. This is usually quite obvious and this change in **vascular territory** is a sensible place to resect proximally.

Whilst you've completely separated off the greater omentum on the right hand side, it's still attached to the proximal greater curvature, so **divide the omentum** right up to your previously chosen **resection level** and do the same thing on the lesser curvature of the stomach with the lesser omentum. The stomach that you want to excise is now **free from any attachments**. Make sure the **nasogastric tube** isn't lying across the resection level! Take a **linear stapling device** and staple across the stomach at your chosen level (the stapler we use in the video also then requires you to cut the stomach off from the stapler but

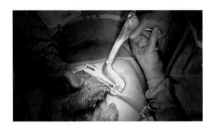

The stapler is applied to the proximal resection margin.

some staplers will run separate rows of staples and cut in between, as for the usual stapling devices used elsewhere). Send the stomach specimen to the **histopathologists**.

Now all that remains is to form a conduit for food to get from the stomach remnant to the jejunum. There are a number of ways of doing this and we demonstrate in this video a hand-sewn anastomosis.

Identify some suitable jejunum by running your hands up and down the small bowel. You want firstly to identify the **ligament of Treitz** superiorly. Lift up the **first loop of jejunum** towards the stomach remnant and make sure it reaches **without any tension**. Hold onto the jejunum with some Babcock forceps and similarly for the stomach. Apply **non-crushing bowel clamps** to the afferent and efferent loops of small bowel and also to the stomach remnant.

Do a **two layer hand-sewn gastro-jejunostomy**, formed by **two concentric circles** of absorbable sutures such

as 2–0 Vicryl. Lay the jejunum next to one half of the stomach staple line. Start by doing the outer layer of sutures. Start at one end of the anastomosis by stitching the **seromuscular layer** of the jejunum to the **seromuscular layer** of the stomach about 1 cm posterior to the staple line. This will be the back wall of the anastomosis. Now **open the stomach** by removing the stapled edge for that half length of the staple line and **open the jejunum** making the hole slightly smaller than the opening in the stomach, but leave a cuff of jejunum between the enterotomy and the seromuscular stitch layer. Now to insert the **back wall of the inner layer** of sutures; start at the same place—the needle should pass through the mucosa of the stomach, the wall of the stomach, the wall of the jejunum and then the mucosa of the jejunum—**all four layers** need to be stitched. Run this suture all around the back wall of the anastomosis and then continue it around the front wall and tie it where you started. Lastly, complete the outer layer by running the seromuscular stitch round the front and tying it where it started. There is a potential site of weakness at the angle between jejunum and stomach ('the angle of sorrow') and a **reinforcing stitch** here is a sensible manoeuvre. That stitch can then be run along the length of the remaining staple line on the stomach for added reinforcement.

With all that completed, **check the duodenal stump** looks healthy and isn't bleeding. **Washout** the abdomen and **close up** in the usual way.

Notes

Of course, not all perforated peptic ulcers require a gastrectomy. We weren't fortunate enough to video one but the principles of repairing them isn't too complex. For either a perforated duodenal ulcer or gastric ulcer, simply stitching the perforation closed isn't enough—the edges of the tissue are inflamed and often friable. It is best therefore to wrap a segment of omentum over the perforation and stitch this in place, putting the stitches some way from the perforation where the wall is healthier. This is an **omental patch repair**.

Moving slightly off the topic of gastrectomies, the other relatively uncommon but zlife-threatening upper gastrointestinal emergency is a **bleeding duodenal ulcer**. We make reference to this in the video and show where you would enter the duodenum. The important thing is to identify the pylorus as described above. You then want to make a longitudinal **gastroduodenotomy** cutting right across the pylorus. You will then typically see the ulcer on the back wall of the first part of the duodenum where it has eroded through into the **gastroduodenal artery;** you may see it hosing from here. Remember this artery is going vertically behind the duodenum, so with some good retraction and sucking from your assistant, stitch transversely just above the bleeding point and then with the same suture make a transverse stitch inferior to the bleeding point, making a **Z shape**. Tie the two ends together. This should stop the bleeding. If not, your stitch wasn't deep enough, or there is a branch of the vessel running in transversely, so repeat the same Z stitch but at 90 degrees to the first, so any vessel running behind that ulcer will be ligated. Be careful with this tissue though, it's often extremely friable and if you tear it you'll end up with nothing to stitch. Once you've achieved haemostasis, close the gastroduodenotomy, not as you opened it as this would result in narrowing of the pylorus, but instead stitch one end of the gastroduodenotomy opening to the other end, thus converting length into width (a **pyloroplasty**). Do two layers and insert a drain.

Pyloroplasty

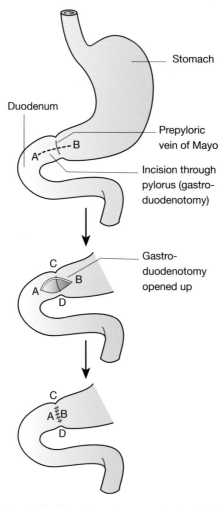

Stomach

Duodenum

Prepyloric vein of Mayo

Incision through pylorus (gastro-duodenotomy)

Gastro-duodenotomy opened up

A gastroduodenotomy is an incision through the pylorus extending into the duodenum and stomach. It's used to access bleeding duodenal ulcers. It's closed in this manner, a pyloroplasty, to prevent pyloric stenosis.

Summary

- The patient is **supine** under **general anaesthetic**
- **Shave, prep** and **drape** the abdomen
- Make an **upper midline laparotomy**
- **Examine** the **abdominal contents** for spread of malignancy
- **Open the lesser sac** via the omentum
- **Feel** between **stomach and pancreas**
- Fully **divide** the right side of the **omentum** of colon
- Ligate and divide the **right gastro-epiploic artery**
- Ligate and divide the **right gastric artery**
- **Divide the duodenum** with a stapler
- Choose the **proximal resection margin**
- **Divide** the **greater omentum** and **lesser omentum** up to this level
- **Staple** across the stomach and **send** to the **histopathologists**
- **Identify** a loop of **jejunum**
- Perform a **hand-sewn two-layer gastrojejunostomy**
- **Reinforce** staple line with **suture**
- Check the **duodenal stump, washout** and **close**

26 Splenectomy

Matt Stephenson and Don Manifold

> **Video** | **15 min 21 s**
> Don Manifold, Consultant General and Upper
> GI Surgeon
> Royal Sussex County Hospital, Brighton

Introduction

The first time you were (or will be) shown how to systematically explore the abdominal contents during a laparotomy, blindly probing with your hand into the depths of the left upper quadrant, the spleen is that organ where you nodded your head sagely and pretended to be able to feel. Measuring on average only **3 x 5 x 7 inches** and lying under **ribs 9 to 11** (**3, 5, 7, 9, 11**) it is a little out of the way. With some practise, you will in fact be able to discriminate it from Gerota's fascia over the kidney, the stomach, the splenic flexure, the diaphragm, a nasogastric tube etc.

Most elective splenectomies however are performed for much larger, and therefore more easily seen and felt, spleens—as evidenced in the video. Many smaller spleens (and not so small spleens) are now being removed laparoscopically.

The **elective indications** are mainly:

- **Hypersplenism**, that is the spleen is overactive resulting in anaemia, leucopenia or thrombocytopenia with consequent bone marrow hyperplasia (strictly speaking, by definition these parameters then have to improve after splenectomy, that's the only way you truly know the spleen was responsible). For instance, in autoimmune conditions (e.g. idiopathic thrombocytopenic purpura), genetic conditions (e.g. hereditary spherocytosis) or haemoglobinopathies (e.g. Sickle cell).
- **Malignancy**, which may be of the lymphoreticular system (e.g. lymphoma) or non-lymphoreticular (e.g. secondaries or direct extension from adjacent malignancies).
- **Diagnostic**, for very large spleens where no other cause can be found, as in our video.
- Rarely, **splenic abscesses**, which can usually be treated with percutaneous drainage, and have a considerable mortality, mainly because they tend to affect the immunocompromised.
- More rarely, very large symptomatic **splenic cysts** and **splenic vein thrombosis**.

How to Operate: for MRCS Candidates and Surgical Trainees, First Edition. M. Stephenson. © 2011 John Wiley & Sons, Ltd.
Published 2011 by John Wiley & Sons, Ltd.

The **emergency indications** are either for:

- **Trauma**—it's a surprisingly easy organ to injure, even in seemingly quite benign blunt trauma—especially if it's already enlarged due to something else (think young people who are recovering from glandular fever playing contact sports (and not the kind that gave them the glandular fever)). More commonly now, however, these injuries are managed conservatively with a careful inpatient watch and wait policy, and this depends on the clinical state of the patient, the haemoglobin and the CT severity grading of the splenic injury (usually Grade I–II conservative, Grade III–V splenectomy but this is contentious).

- **Iatrogenic**—most commonly during mobilisation of the splenic flexure of the colon— pulling too hard here will tear the attachments which are firmly adherent to the capsule. If swab pressure doesn't stop it, the spleen will have to come out.

Never forget, of course, that these patients must have their **vaccinations** against organisms of the encapsulated variety: *Haemophilus influenzae, Streptococcus pneumoniae* and *Neisseria meningitides*. Ideally, this should be at least 4–6 weeks before surgery. In the emergency setting, waiting about 2 weeks to allow the patient to get over the surgery will increase the effectiveness of the vaccine. **Prophylactic antibiotics**, however, must be started in both groups immediately, usually in the form of penicillin V, which most people believe should be taken lifelong. The patient must then always avoid areas at risk of **malaria** and carry **information** on their person about their splenectomised state.

Procedure

The patient is **supine** under **general anaesthetic**. A **urinary catheter** and **nasogastric tube** are *in situ*. Perioperative **antibiotics** have been given. The two options are an **upper midline incision** or a **left costal incision**. The left subcostal is basically the mirror image of the Kocher's scar described in the *Open Cholecystectomy* Chapter 28, so it won't be repeated here. In general, choose the left subcostal incision for smaller spleens and the midline for larger ones. Going in through the midline enables you to access the splenic artery some way distant from the spleen and get control of it in case there's a lot of bleeding from

the spleen. Always go midline for trauma situations. So whatever your access, the rest of the operation is the same.

Pick up the stomach and note the omentum hanging down from it over the transverse colon. Enter the **lesser sac** here by **opening the gastrocolic omentum** between these two. For a long discussion about the lesser sac—read the *Gastrectomy* Chapter 25. So you've made a window in the omentum and you'll be able to see the back wall of the **stomach** and the **pancreas** behind that. You're on the look out for the **splenic artery** which usually runs over the **superior surface** of the pancreas. Sometimes you need to divide some adhesions between the

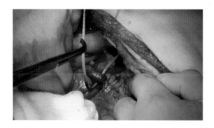

The splenic artery is seen with a sloop around it. Just inferior is the pancreas and the stomach reflected away above.

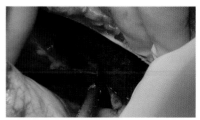

To the left is the stomach being retracted medially and the spleen is seen to the right. The Harmonic scalpel is divided the gastrosplenic ligament between them, in there are the short gastric arteries.

stomach and the pancreas. Once you find the artery running more or less transversely (but can be very tortuous) over the top of the pancreas, **dissect around it gently**, bearing in mind it will have small side branches going off into the pancreas. Get right angled forceps, like **Lahey's**, around it and **double sling it** with a vascular sloop—pulling up on this now will dramatically reduce the blood flow to the spleen, having the effect of **shrinking** a very large spleen to help in dissection, or just being able to **control the blood flow** if you make a nick in the splenic capsule. Leave that like that for now and begin the splenectomy—which is essentially just a matter of **dividing all of its attachments**. You can do this division with traditional ligating and dividing, diathermy, Harmonic scalpel or a combination of these.

You've already opened the gastrocolic omentum to find the proximal splenic artery (and if you didn't do this step, open the omentum now). If you follow the omentum up around the greater curvature of the stomach, it becomes the **gastro-splenic ligament**. Therefore continue to

divide it, but keep away from the stomach to avoid damaging that vascular arcade. You'll see the stomach then to the left and the spleen to the right with the gastro-splenic ligament being divided in between, and in it are the **short gastric arteries** running north from the splenic artery to feed the stomach—**divide them** carefully here as they run too close to the spleen and the splenic hilum to preserve them.

Usually the next step that's easiest to undertake is the **inferior attachments** (the **splenocolic ligament**) of the spleen down to the splenic flexure of the colon. Push the bowel inferiorly, packing it away with a

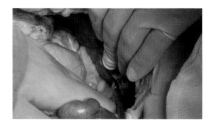

The Harmonic scalpel is dividing the inferior attachments of the spleen.

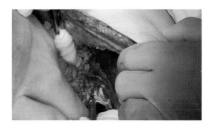

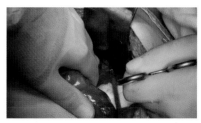

The splenic vein is revealed inside, the inferior pole vessels are being divided.

The spleen is now being pulled medially and the lateral abdominal wall retracted laterally to see the lienorenal ligament.

swab may help, and retract the spleen superiorly. Take care with these attachments—**cut them, don't tear them**.

You can then divide the **peritoneum overlying the splenic hilum**. Beneath it you'll find the **splenic artery** and the **splenic vein**—or you may find **several branches** of each. Try to **divide the smaller branches** feeding the superior and inferior poles of the spleen. This will have the effect of making the spleen tethered only to the main central vessels and when it comes to delivering it, it will be hanging only from a fairly thin central leash. You can, if you'd prefer, divide all these big vessels now as well, but it comes with a higher risk of **damaging the tail of the pancreas**, the tip of which mingles with the splenic hilum. If you wait until later and the spleen is fully delivered, it's easier to see the pancreas in relation to those vessels.

So all that remains is to divide the **lienorenal ligament** attaching the spleen laterally to Gerota's fascia over the kidney and then follow that superiorly to the upper portion of the **phrenicocolic**

ligament, also called the **sustentaculum lienis** which 'suspends' the spleen from the diaphragm. It sometimes helps to tilt the table toward you slightly. These have the name 'ligament', but they are really just **condensations of peritoneum**, and are therefore quite easy to cut through. Sometimes you can see this part of the operation under clear direct vision (the lienorenal ligament is, you'll be pleased to hear, relatively avascular). Sometimes however, it has to be done blindly by feel alone, which at first can seem a bit daunting—reaching up into the depths of the left upper quadrant snipping away with a pair of long scissors feeling the patient's heart beating away against the diaphragm superiorly. You may find it more daunting doing this in the emergency situation when the wound keeps welling up with blood.

With all these attachments freed up, you can **deliver the spleen** out into the wound where it is attached only by that leash of vessels and here in better light you can **divide the splenic artery first** (to allow the spleen time to drain) by either

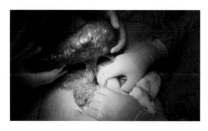

The spleen has been delivered out of the wound, attached only by the major vessels.

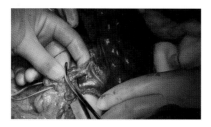

The splenic artery has been ligated, the splenic vein is next.

double ligation with a strong tie, or transfixion. The same can then be done for the **splenic vein**. If you put a sling around the splenic artery at the beginning, don't forget to now remove it! Make sure you **check the splenic hilar area for splenunculi**, found in around 10% of patients. In emergency situations, leave these be—the patient could do with a bit of accessory splenic tissue. Most elective situations though mandate that these are also removed.

With the spleen removed and sent to **histopathology**, check the wound bed for **bleeding**, which is usually from the cut edge of peritoneum. **Wash out the wound** to remove any bits of clot that can act as a nidus for infection. Consider inserting a **drain** if it's been particularly oozy or you're worried there may be an injury to the pancreatic tail. In general leave the nasogastric tube in for 24 hours, as there is often a gastric ileus since you've been handling it. **Close the wound** in the usual **mass closure** way.

Notes

There is **no absolute order** in which to do these steps. If it seems easier for instance to approach the splenic hilum before the inferior attachments, or mobilise the spleen earlier by first dividing the lienorenal ligaments or the short gastrics before the proximal splenic artery isolation (as in the video), there's no law against it. Do whatever seems to be the next natural step, basically just detach the spleen from everything around it.

Some surgeons, when isolating that segment of proximal splenic artery through the lesser sac, rather than just putting a vascular sloop around it, will formally ligate it (there's no need to actually divide it). Some will then also inject 1 ml of 1 : 10 000 adrenaline into the artery in an effort to vasoconstrict the spleen.

In the **trauma situation**, the bleeding can be a real issue, especially if the major hilar vessels have been avulsed (a grade V injury). On entering the abdomen and sucking out the blood—pack the left upper quadrant firmly with large swabs in an attempt to tamponade the bleeding whilst you isolate the splenic artery through the lesser sac. Much of the operation must then still be done blindly by holding the spleen in your non-dominant hand and cutting the attachments around it with scissors, by feel. The first sensible step in these scenarios is to pull the spleen medially and divide the lienorenal ligament, thus mobilising it; this may be possible bluntly with your fingers. It may also help to pinch the splenic hilum between finger and thumb.

Be aware that not all splenic injuries, even if you've operated on them, need a splenectomy. If the bleeding is from one point and has easily been controlled with pressure and a haemostatic agent like Surgicel—consider leaving the spleen in the patient and monitoring them carefully postoperatively. If you do need to do a splenectomy, you might even consider leaving thin slices of spleen embedded in the omentum in the hope they grow and return some splenic function—so called **conservative splenic surgery**.

Summary

- Preoperative **vaccinations** have been given if possible and all have perioperative **antibiotics**
- The patient is **supine** and under **general anaesthetic**
- Make an **upper midline** or **left subcostal** incision
- Isolate the proximal part of the **splenic artery** through the **lesser sac** if appropriate
- Divide the **short gastric arteries** in the **gastrosplenic ligament**
- Divide the inferior attachments, the **splenocolic ligament**
- Divide the **peritoneum over the hilum** and the **upper and lower pole vessels**
- Divide the **lienorenal ligament** and the **sustentaculum lienis**
- **Deliver the spleen**
- Ligate and divide the **splenic artery then vein**
- Check for **splenunculi**
- Send to **histopathology**
- Check for **bleeding**
- Consider **lavage** and **drains**
- Perform a **mass closure** (for either incision)
- Make sure the patient is written up for **antibiotics**

27 Gastrojejunostomy

Matt Stephenson and Peter C Hale

> **Video** | **11 min 20 s**
> Peter C Hale, Consultant General and Upper GI Surgeon
> Royal Sussex County Hospital, Brighton

Introduction

It's 3 o'clock in the morning and you've taken your patient to theatre for a laparotomy for an acute abdomen and discover a massive **duodenal ulcer** that's perforated and left the duodenum a ragged inflamed mess, completely unsuitable as a conduit for food to pass through even if you try and repair it. Or imagine you've taken the patient for a laparotomy for, say, a clinical diagnosis of bowel obstruction, the CT was pretty non-specific. You discover an obstructing **gastric outlet lesion** stuck firmly to the back of the pancreas (perhaps somebody could have taken a better history). If you try and resect it off it will bleed and bleed and you'll regret trying. What are you going to do? The **gastro-jejunostomy** is your **get out of jail free card**. In the former example it reduces the risk of a blown duodenum, in the latter it provides palliation for the patient. It can also be the way you re-plumb the gastric remnant onto the jejunum after a partial gastrectomy.

It is therefore an extremely important skill for any general surgeon, and fortunately for you it's really no more difficult than a standard small bowel anastomosis as long as you understand the key aspects we'll show here.

There is much debate about whether gastrojejunostomies should be (1) **hand sewn** or **stapled**, (2) **antecolic** or **retrocolic**, or (3) **isoperistaltic** or **antiperistaltic**.

Firstly, at 3 o'clock in the morning a stapled anastomosis is much **quicker** and **equally effective** as a hand-sewn one. Secondly, antecolic means that you bring up the loop of jejunum to the **anterior surface** of the stomach whereas retrocolic means that you lift up the omentum and transverse colon and enter the lesser sac through a hole you make in the back of the transverse mesocolon and anastomose it onto the back of the stomach. The former is usually far easier for the junior surgeon, so stick to what you can safely do. Thirdly, an isoperistaltic anastomosis means that the loop of jejunum is in the **same direction** as the stomach, antiperistaltic means the loop of jejunum is twisted

How to Operate: for MRCS Candidates and Surgical Trainees, First Edition. M. Stephenson. © 2011 John Wiley & Sons, Ltd.
Published 2011 by John Wiley & Sons, Ltd.

round, so in the other direction. This is really only for revision gastrojejunostomies in cases of dumping, for instance, and you want to slow down gastric emptying.

So keep it simple: antecolic, isoperistaltic, stapled gastrojejunostomy.

Procedure

You may have been planning to do a gastrojejunostomy preoperatively if, for instance, preoperative imaging was highly suggestive of an inoperable tumour of the gastric outlet. Alternatively it may come as an unpleasant surprise, so you'll have to be adaptable. But we can assume that the patient is **supine** under **general anaesthetic** with an **upper midline laparotomy** wound and that you have already examined the abdominal contents and arrived at the decision that a gastrojejunostomy is the best option.

So you need to **prepare** your two bits of gut for anastomosis. Firstly, **draw the stomach down** in to your wound by applying two non-crushing forceps like **Duval's** along the greater curvature of the stomach some distance apart. Make sure that the area of stomach between your forceps is: (1) **proximal to tumour**

(too close and it will close up quickly from further cancerous growth); (2) the **anterior surface** of stomach; and (3) ideally the **most dependent part** of the stomach. Leave the stomach there like that for now.

Next you need a **loop of jejunum** for anastomosis. Deliver all of the small bowel out for examination. **Trace it up** all the way proximally to the **duodenojejunal flexure** which is held up by the **ligament of Treitz**. Now trace it back distally until you get far enough along jejunum that it will **easily flop up** to greet the bit of stomach you've prepared **without any tension**. As you have with the stomach, hold the jejunum between two non-crushing forceps like **Babcock's**, on the **antimesenteric border**—the area in between will be the surface for anastomosis. Bring **stomach and jejunum together** and make sure there is **no tension**.

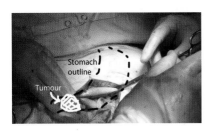

The underlying position of the stomach and tumour has been outlined.

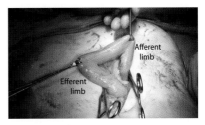

The proximal jejunum has been mobilised and is held between Babcock forceps.

Lay swabs around the wound edge to **reduce contamination**. Make a **small hole** in the stomach and one on the jejunum at a corresponding position between the forceps, these will be for the jaws of the **linear stapler**. You can use diathermy for this but when you get through to the mucosa, it's best to cut this with scissors as it's too easy to go straight through to the other wall with the diathermy, thus injuring it. The hole can be pretty small, the stapler stretches them up. Remember also that the afferent loop of jejunum is going up to the anastomosis and the efferent loop is leaving it. What you really don't want is for the anastomosis to be narrowed at the efferent end (although you don't want it narrowed at either end). **Stenosis** can occur where you later stitch up these two holes; therefore, make the holes at the **afferent end** of the anastomosis, a stenosis at the afferent end is more inconsequential (but can still be a big problem).

Insert each jaw of the stapler into the holes and bring the stomach and jejunum together and allow the stapler jaws to **engage** with each other. Take care that you're getting the **antimesenteric border** of the jejunum and that nothing has been **trapped** in the stapler behind, or

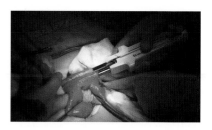

The stapler has been inserted; note the finger below the line of staples checking nothing else wants to get in on the action.

that the **nasogastric tube** isn't going to be included. Push the **sliding mechanism** of the stapler forward thus making **two rows** of staples, then slide it back, which **cuts** between the two rows. **Remove the stapler** and all that remains is to **close the stapler hole**. Close this with a continuous **full thickness layer** of absorbable suture such as 2–0 Vicryl followed by a **continuous seromuscular layer** which inverts the first layer. Check the **patency** of the anastomosis between finger and thumb—ideally it should be able to admit about two fingers, although obviously you have to estimate this from the outside.

Close up in the usual way with mass closure.

Summary

- Establish that a gastrojejunostomy is the **right operation**, this may be intraoperative
- Hold the **anterior stomach** with two **non-crushing forceps** and draw it down into the wound
- **Deliver** the small bowel into the wound and trace up to the **ligament of Treitz**
- Find the **first part of the jejunum** which comes up to meet the stomach **without tension**
- Hold on to this with **non-crushing forceps**
- **Bring the two together**
- Make a **small hole** in each
- **Insert the jaws** of the linear stapler
- **Staple and cut** by using the sliding mechanism on the stapler
- **Close up the defect** with absorbable suture
- Check the **patency**

28 Open Cholecystectomy

Matt Stephenson and Peter C Hale

> **Video** | **8 min 55 s**
> Peter C Hale, Consultant General and Upper GI Surgeon
> Royal Sussex County Hospital, Brighton

Introduction

Given the ubiquity of the laparoscopic cholecystectomy it's hardly surprising that open cholecystectomies have become something of a rarity these days. So much so in fact that, anecdotally, many registrars may reach the end of their training having done a meagre handful. In the olden days, they were as common as the open appendicectomy— also of course now an endangered species. But this is a worrying state of affairs—anyone doing a laparoscopic cholecystectomy **must** also be able to do it open. If things go wrong laparoscopically you need a plan B and that means opening the patient and seeing and feeling everything properly in three dimensions. The problem of course is increased by the fact that if you do need to convert to open, or even start open because you're anticipating a hostile abdomen in the case of multiple previous operations for instance— then by definition these are going to be the hardest gallbladders to safely take out! And they can be really difficult, and with the bile ducts so nearby, the stakes are high. Without some practise on some easy ones you are therefore at quite a disadvantage.

Hopefully however, this chapter and video will give you a clear idea of how it's done, and then when the opportunity arises in theatre—hopefully your boss will give it to you. Bear in mind that ordinarily you would do this operation through a **right subcostal** (or **Kocher's**) incision. Our patient for the video was also having a repair of a large paraoesophageal hernia and exploration of the bile ducts at the same time—hence the open operation with a midline scar. We'll explain the Kocher's incision however—it's very straightforward and hopefully this explanation will be enough although the transverse incision for the *Right Hemicolectomy* video is identical in the layers to go through, just a different angle.

How to Operate: for MRCS Candidates and Surgical Trainees, First Edition. M. Stephenson. © 2011 John Wiley & Sons, Ltd.
Published 2011 by John Wiley & Sons, Ltd.

As a little bonus, we've included a brief bit on exploration of the bile ducts as this patient was having it anyway. It's not a comprehensive 'how to do a bile exploration' (partly because it was so difficult to film down that dark hole), but it's a little taster and may help understand what T-tubes are all about.

Procedure

With the patient **supine** under **general anaesthetic, prep** and **drape** the whole of the upper abdomen. **Palpate** the lower border of the right costal margin and make an incision about **2 or 3 cm below** it from about the **midline** to about the **anterior axillary line**. If you've just converted from a laparoscopic operation, then try to **include the port holes** in the incision if they're not too far off.

Incise through **skin**, **superficial fascia** and **fat** down to the **anterior rectus sheath**. Incise straight down to reveal the vertical fibres of **rectus abdominus**. Laterally there is the **external oblique aponeurosis**, **cut** straight through this in continuity with the anterior rectus sheath. Gently pass a **long clip underneath** the rectus abdominus, under the lateral border and coming out at the midline between the two recti. Get hold of a **nylon tape** or the tassel of a swab in the clip and pull this through and **pull upwards** on the tape (or tassel). The rectus abdominus is now being held up by the tape. Have your assistant take hold of one end of it and you take the other. Using finger-switch diathermy, slowly **divide** the muscle transversely as it's being tented up by the nylon tape. Bear in mind the **superior epigastric artery** will

be in it along with some other branches. Try to diathermy these before the ends retract into the muscle and keep bleeding until your boss decides you're not up to it and takes over your precious operation. Once you've divided rectus, you're up against **posterior rectus sheath** with **peritoneum** underneath. **Laterally**, **divide** the external oblique, internal oblique and transversus in the line of the incision. **Pick up** the posterior rectus sheath with **two clips**, **feel** between finger and thumb that nothing's adherent to the back of it and open with scissors. With the peritoneum open, **sweep** a finger inside to check for adhesions and providing all's safe **divide** the posterior rectus sheath and peritoneum, and whatever's left laterally with diathermy in the line of the wound.

So far, the operation is easiest to perform from the **right side**. Once you're into the abdomen however, some people like to continue with the operation from the **left hand** side thus attacking the gallbladder from across the table, it's all how you're brought up and either is fine as long as you're comfortable doing it. In the video, it's being done from the right.

Fingers crossed, right beneath your wound will be a liver edge with a **little pink dome** peeping out from underneath—this is probably the gallbladder although don't mistake the **hepatic flexure** of colon for it, which has been done—it's obvious if you look carefully. If you're unlucky, you'll find a mass of **omentum** all stuck up to the right upper quadrant completely concealing the gallbladder. If so, carefully **dissect it off the liver**, usually using blunt dissection, until the gallbladder comes into view. This part is quite easy, you're unlucky because it's a bad omen of things to come—Calot's triangle is also likely to be inflamed and treacherous, but not necessarily.

The first step of the cholecystectomy, apart from finding the gallbladder, is getting **control** of it. This is best achieved by using a **Rampley sponge holder**, which is non-crushing and clasps it over a large surface area. The lower down on the gallbladder you can get hold of it the better so ideally you want it on **Hartmann's pouch**. You can now pull up on the sponge holder gently thus drawing it up towards your wound but also, mainly, laterally. This will **open out Calot's triangle** which is the key to this operation—a quick reminder of what the borders are: **cystic duct**, **common hepatic duct** and **liver edge**, and it usually contains the **cystic artery** (actually Calot described the sides of the triangle as the cystic duct, common hepatic duct and cystic artery—so if Calot got his own triangle wrong you can be forgiven if it slipped your memory . . .). Your assistant, standing on the other side needs to use his or her hand to retract the small bowel.

Imagine you're standing on the patient's right. In your left hand is the sponge holder controlling the gallbladder. You're looking more or less **vertically down** onto Calot's triangle. It's a slightly different angle than you may be used to with the laparoscopic view, and much **less magnified**. With your right hand **palpate** the gallbladder for stones feeling your way down the gallbladder to Calot's triangle. Is it all swollen and indurated? Then you're in for a time of it, the dissection may be very difficult and the planes unclear (see Notes below). If it's fairly thin and mobile you're in luck. Either way, the next thing to do with your right hand is to carefully **dissect** off the layer of **peritoneum** covering Calot's triangle. A good way of doing this is pull up and laterally with the sponge holder in the palm of your hand with your fingertips each side of the gallbladder and the safest place to start is the most inferior edge of peritoneum. Just **nibble** at it with the **tips of your scissors** and open it up in a **line** close to the gallbladder up toward the liver. Hopefully, once the peritoneum is

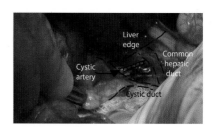

The borders of Calot's triangle have been outlined and labelled.

opened, the less robust connective tissue within will **separate out** giving you a view of a tube in continuity with the gallbladder heading medially—this may be the **cystic duct**, but you don't know yet, but if it is, it's one side of the sacred triangle.

Keeping close to the gallbladder, dissect out between it and the liver until you've carefully examined the whole of that space. How do you dissect it? Everyone has their preferences but most people use a combination of **blunt dissection** with **pledgets** and **fingers**, and **sharp dissection** with **scissors** and the **judicious** use of the **diathermy** (short bursts only here and as low energy as possible—heat travels to neighbouring tissues easily and late strictures of the common hepatic duct are a recognised complication). So once you've dissected up to the liver edge, you've got two sides to the triangle. What about the third, the common hepatic duct? Well you don't actually have to dissect that out, it can be unnecessarily dangerous. The purpose of dissecting out the triangle is to make sure that you aren't accidentally ligating the common hepatic duct or similar by mistaking it for the cystic duct. If you've dissected all the way up the edge of the liver and confirm there is only one tube (or occasionally two) going in to the gallbladder, and that definitely isn't going near it and then skirting off again (a favourite trick of the suicidal common hepatic duct), then you can **safely divide it**. It also helps you find the cystic artery, which will be somewhere within all that tissue.

So ligate and **divide the cystic artery first**, some use a suture, some use ligaclips. Then ligate and divide the cystic duct, transfixing it is safer. Always do the

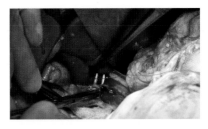

The Lahey forceps are hooked around the cystic artery to ligate it.

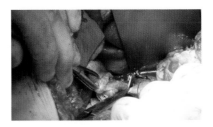

The cystic duct has been clipped with Lahey forceps and it's about to be transfixed.

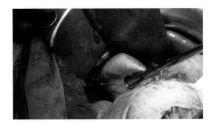

The fundus of the gallbladder has been retracted medially and the plane between it and liver is exposed to be divided.

artery first, if you do the cystic duct first, the traction on the gallbladder **can easily tear** the less robust cystic artery. Once you've got those two divided, you can pull up fairly firmly on the sponge holder and **put tension** on the tissue holding the gallbladder to its fossa. **Diathermy** between the two—there is usually a plane between gallbladder and liver, it will help to **move the sponge holder** to different places on the gallbladder to get sufficient tension, and often moving back up to the fundus at this point helps. Keep an eye out for any **accessory ducts** draining straight across from the gallbladder fossa which will continuously ooze bile over the next few days (meaning the patient will need a drain, endoscopic retrograde cholangiopancreatography (ERCP) and possible reoperation). It often **bleeds** substantially (especially if you get into the wrong plane), but curiously almost always stops once the gallbladder is off. Some firm, prolonged pressure on the fossa with a **swab on a stick** (those Rampley sponge holders must have been made for this operation) will help for those more disobedient ones.

Always look down at the end into the remnant of Calot's triangle to check your clips, ties or sutures look secure and that it's not welling up with **blood or bile**. **Wash** it out if there was any bilious contamination. **Drains** are contentious. **Close** all the layers of the abdominal wall in one, as with the midline **mass closure** and close the skin with **subcuticular** absorbable suture.

Notes

This operation can be really quite **difficult** at times, but there are a number of tricks that can help.

Sometimes the gallbladder is so **distended** and the wall so **thickened**, you can't get any purchase on it with your sponge holder. Take a green needle and syringe and **aspirate** as much bile as you can (if currently infected send it for microbiological assessment) and it should become easier to get hold of. If the gallbladder is packed with stones giving the same problem, you can simply **open it** and take all the stones out.

The most hazardous scenario is if you're struggling to dissect out Calot's triangle, because of very **oedematous** tissues (in the case of the hot gallbladder) and **adhesions** and subsequent **loss of normal anatomy** and difficulties in **identifying the planes** and structures. Alternatively the patient may simply have an **abnormal anatomical configuration**. The first thing you can try is dissecting the gallbladder off the liver bed starting **from the fundus** ('fundus first') and working your way down towards Calot's triangle from that different approach. In the worst case scenario and it's simply not safe to proceed without risking damage to the bile ducts, **open the gallbladder** as low as you safely can by cutting straight across it thus removing most of the gallbladder. **Drain any bile** and manually **remove any stones** in the remnant. You should then be able to **identify the internal opening** of the cystic duct, which should help you to then dissect off the gallbladder remnant safely knowing at least where that is. However, if you can't safely identify the cystic duct to ligate it, there's no shame in calling it quits and sewing up the gallbladder remnant as low as you can on Hartmann's pouch— a **subtotal cholecystectomy**.

Lastly regarding **T-tubes**, which often seem to be a bit of a mystery to the uninitiated. Whenever you open the bile ducts, either to explore them or by accident (if for instance the common hepatic duct was torn from excessive traction on the cystic duct), you have to decide if you want to **close the duct primarily** or **insert a T-tube**. You might wonder why you would ever want to not simply close the tube with a stitch, surely that's less hassle? The problem mainly is that the tube is very narrow already and closing a defect in it with stitches is necessarily going to narrow it further, resulting in the risk of a late **biliary stricture**. Not only this, but if the pressure in the duct breaks open the defect again despite your meticulous stitching you then have a bile leak on your hands. By inserting a T-tube, with one end of the head of the T going up towards the liver, the other end down towards the ampulla and the tail out into a drainage bag, you are creating a controlled communication between bile ducts and a drainage bag. It closes the defect, drains any bile (preventing it leaking) whilst still allowing most of it go down through the duct the natural way, and also provides a useful means of examining the ducts at a later date via a **T-tube cholangiogram**, which is a useful way of confirming there are no residual stones. If you leave the T-tube *in situ* for about a month, an epithelialising lining will be developing all around it, which means that you can remove it and you're left with a **fistula** between bile duct and skin. After a month therefore you can remove the T-tube confident the bile won't leak out of the duct it will go down the track formed by the T-tube out into a drainage bag stuck on the skin. That fistula will then close up with time provided there is no distal obstruction to the common bile duct. In the video you will see the bile ducts being explored using a **choledochoscope** which visualises the inside of the ducts. If a stone is found it can be retrieved using special forceps or a special trawler.

Summary

- The patient is **supine** under **general anaesthetic**
- The abdomen is **prepped** and **draped** to expose the right upper quadrant
- Make a **right subcostal incision**
- **Incise** through **skin, superficial fascia** and **fat**
- Cut through **anterior rectus sheath** and **external oblique**
- Divide the **rectus abdominus** muscle
- Open **peritoneum**

(Continued)

- **Grasp Hartmann's pouch** and retract the small bowel to create space
- **Dissect the peritoneum** over Calot's triangle
- Identify **cystic artery** and **duct**
- When confident you know the anatomy **ligate** and **divide** the **cystic artery**
- **Transfix the cystic duct** and divide
- **Dissect** off the **gallbladder fossa**
- Establish **haemostasis** and **check the clips** remain where they should
- Close all the layers in a **mass closure** with **subcuticular absorbable** suture to skin

29 Thoracotomy

Matt Stephenson and Don Manifold

> **Video** | **11 min 0 s**
> Don Manifold, Consultant General and
> Upper GI Surgeon
> Royal Sussex County Hospital, Brighton

Introduction

There are a variety of approaches through the chest wall to access the thoracic contents. They could be generally divided into midline, lateral or a combination of both. All of the lateral approaches being through intercostal spaces, but varying in which intercostal space and whether they extend more posteriorly or anteriorly.

1 Median sternotomy: a midline incision and then division of the sternum longitudinally from top to bottom and retracting each side of the rib cage laterally to access the heart or superior mediastinum. Clearly more cardiothoracic territory then.

2 Clamshell thoracotomy: used rarely and only in the true emergency scenario in cardiac arrests of the pulseless electrical activity (PEA) variety in the presence of penetrating thoracic trauma. The kind of operation you'll only ever read or hear about in heroic tales before you might be in the situation where you'll need to use it yourself, and then maybe only once in a career. You make bilateral anterolateral thoracotomies that meet in the middle by cutting through the sternum allowing you to lift up the whole upper chest wall like a clamshell to access the whole thoracic cavity.

3 Posterolateral: the standard route of access to the posterior mediastinum. The incision begins about 7.5 cm lateral to the midspinal line round the back and courses round the inferior tip of the scapula to the anterior axillary line going usually through about the 5th or 6th intercostal space.

4 Anterolateral: can be used on the left side for emergency access to the heart in the presence of penetrating injuries. The incision is through the 4th or 5th intercostal spaces

5 Left lateral: for access to the lower oesophagus via the left 7th intercostal space—featured in this video. On the right you would access the oesophagus via a right posterolateral thoracotomy.

How to Operate: for MRCS Candidates and Surgical Trainees, First Edition. M. Stephenson. © 2011 John Wiley & Sons, Ltd.
Published 2011 by John Wiley & Sons, Ltd.

6 Thoracoabdominal: for operations requiring adequate exposure to the hiatus—some oesophageal and gastric resections, splenectomy where the diaphragm may be involved and revisional antireflux surgery. The midline laparotomy turns from its superior end towards the 4th or 5th intercostal space on the left (higher than a pure thoracotomy approach to the oesophagus as you can already access the lower oesophagus transhiatally from the laparotomy).

There are three main reasons a general surgeon might need to open the chest: to operate on the oesophagus, to operate on the thoracic aorta and in the case of thoracic trauma.

The patient in the video had a suspected Boerhaave's syndrome so access to the lower oesophagus was needed, hence a left lateral thoracotomy. However, the principles of the procedure are the same across the other approaches, they only really differ in the level of intercostal space and the muscles encountered. In standard approaches to these thoracotomies, you just cut through whatever muscles you encounter as we do here.

Procedure

The patient is in the **left lateral** position with the **body supported** with sandbags and tape where necessary to ensure **stability** and attention to protecting **pressure areas**. **Prep** and **drape** the chest, including dirty areas like the armpit. Since you're unlikely to be as familiar with the patient lying on their side, **identify**

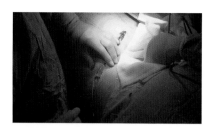

Remember the patient is lying on his side. The surgeon is to the left of the picture with the patient facing away.

some landmarks to help orient you. Find the nipple, the costal margin and the tip of the scapula. The tip of the scapula in the lateral position is around the 5–6th intercostal space posteriorly and the nipple tends to overlie the 4th intercostal space anteriorly. This should help estimate the level of intercostal space to go for.

Make an **incision** through **skin** over the **7th intercostal space** from about the **midclavicular** line to the **posterior axillary** line. Incise through **superficial fascia** and **fat** until you come down onto the fascia overlying muscle. The anterior part of the incision is over **serratus anterior;** further posteriorly, this is overlapped by the anterior edge of **latissimus dorsi**. There is a fascial plane between the serratus anterior and latissimus dorsi. **Cut** through both of these muscles with diathermy in the line of the incision. Make

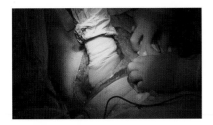

The operating hand is inserted under serratus anterior over the rib cage.

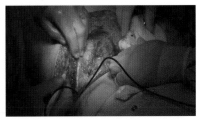

A white rib is seen just next to the surgeon's left hand, the intercostal space is opened just superiorly to this.

sure you catch any larger vessels running in it and give them a good buzz with the diathermy before they retract into the body of the muscle.

You then see **white ribs** appearing and you can now put your **hand up** over the rib cage, deep to serratus anterior and feel the scapula posteriorly and the ribs deeply. The highest one you can feel here is usually the second rib, **count down** the ribs until you find the 7th intercostal space, which hopefully will be roughly the level of your approach anyway.

Some people cut straight through the intercostal muscles, others (as we have in the video) **incise the periosteum** of the rib where those muscles are inserted to lift off the muscles. Either way, since the **neurovascular bundle** runs in the **intercostal groove**, which is on the inferior edge of each rib, clearly you don't want to go too near that, so therefore approach the intercostal space through the **superior edge of the rib below**. Don't incise the inferior edge of the rib above. The same principle of course applies to inserting chest drains in other scenarios.

Lift off or incise with diathermy the **external** and then **internal intercostal** muscles which run perpendicular to each other and are often seen distinctly separately from each other, especially in men compared to women. Deep to that layer you'll find the **pleural lining**—the equivalent of the peritoneal lining in the abdomen. **Puncture** the pleural lining and **insert a finger** to dissect a larger hole in it. Hook it round under the pleural lining and diathermy straight down onto it in the line of the intercostal space to the full extent of the wound.

To open up the cavity it helps to **excise a small segment** of the adjacent rib

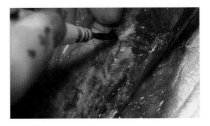

Just below and right of the diathermy point is a window in the intercostal muscles through which the pleural membrane can be seen.

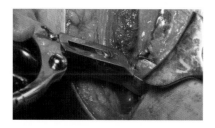

This costotome is excising a small segment of rib.

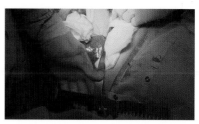

This is a Finnicetto rib retractor opening up the rib space.

above, posteriorly, which then allows the anterior part of the rib to be retracted much more easily. To do this, **divide** the full thickness of the **intercostal muscles** in that space at the chosen point of rib division. This allows you to **insert a costotome** to encircle the rib. Cut it in two places, just a centimetre or so apart and remove the small segment of floating rib.

Now insert a **rib retractor**. Similar to many abdominal retractors, it has **two blades** (of the non-sharp variety) which can be distracted from each other by a **wind up mechanism**, thus allowing quite a significant amount of force to be applied. **Protect the ribs** with swabs and insert the blade component into the space. Wind up the mechanism. If it seems to be taking a lot of strength to wind it up, a rib is probably about to crack. **Pause** for a minute or two and start winding again, it usually allows the muscles to relax and the ribs to part uneventfully. You can then get on with whatever thoracic procedure you were doing—but that's the subject of another book/DVD.

Fast forwarding to the **closure** stages, it's always **mandatory** after a thoracic procedure to **insert a chest drain**—both to drain any postoperative fluid and blood, but also to drain any air that may escape from a damaged lung for instance. Worst case scenario this can lead to a life threatening **tension pneumothorax**. Try to get the tip of the chest drain pointing up to the **apex** of the pleural cavity and bring it out through an intercostal space lower than you entered the chest. Try to bring it out through the skin reasonably anteriorly where it won't be uncomfortable for the patient to lie on.

Close the rib space itself with two or three strong nylon or PDS sutures. Having

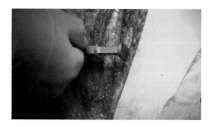

A rib approximator is used to hold the ribs together for ease of tying knots.

stretched the ribs apart, it can be a little difficult to get them to come back together again. If you have one, use a **rib approximator** which holds the rib above and the rib below together allowing you to tie your sutures without them slipping. You don't need to close the intercostal muscles.

Close the deep **serratus anterior** layer with its surrounding fascia with a continuous absorbable suture and then the same for the **latissimus dorsi** and its fascia. If the patient has a thick fat layer you might want to approximate it with another continuous suture with a final continuous subcuticular **absorbable suture to skin**. Apply dressings.

Thoracotomies are one of the most **painful** wounds to recover from. A thoracic epidural can help or an intercostal nerve block, but they may need a significant amount of opiates. Watch the drain output postoperatively; how long it needs to stay in for depends on the procedure you've just done.

Summary

- The patient is under **general anaesthetic**
- Position the patient in the **left lateral** position
- Identify **landmarks** to orient yourself
- **Incise** along the estimated **7th intercostal space**
- Incise through **serratus anterior** and **latissimus dorsi**
- **Palpate over the rib cage** to feel the scapula posteriorly and the rib cage deeply
- **Incise the periosteum** over the rib below the 7th intercostal space
- **Open the pleural** membrane
- **Divide segment of bone** with costotome
- Insert **rib retractor** and retract
- Do the thoracic operation
- Insert a **chest drain**
- **Close** the **intercostal space** with two or three sutures
- **Close** the **serratus anterior** layer
- **Close** the **latissimus dorsi** layer
- **Close skin**

30 Mastectomy

Matt Stephenson and Elizabeth F Shah

> **Video** | **8 min 32 s**
> Elizabeth F Shah, Consultant Oncoplastic Breast Surgeon
> Conquest Hospital, St Leonards-on-Sea

Introduction

Mastectomies have changed over the decades from radical, highly deforming surgery to relatively more conservative (but equally oncologically sound) resection of breast tissue, often with the option of reconstructive surgery. However, a mastectomy can still be a totally **life changing event** for a woman. You as her surgeon not only need to tend to the **emotional aspects** of breast cancer and surgery, but need to do a **meticulous, careful operation**. A high rate of postoperative haematomas, wound infections, necrosed skin flaps, ugly scars and residual oncopotential breast tissue can all be avoided.

Here we describe the **simple mastectomy;** if combined with complete removal of the axillary lymph nodes it's called a **modified radical mastectomy** (or **Patey** mastectomy). What was this modified from? A **radical mastectomy**, or **Halsted mastectomy** (very rarely done now) also meant excising the pectoralis muscles, which was a highly disfiguring operation with no significant oncological advantage; you don't therefore need to know how to do it. If however you found the tumour was penetrating the pectoralis major muscle, it would certainly be appropriate to excise a good margin of pectoralis major muscle with it. This however should have been worked out pre-operatively by clinical examination, and consideration given to the unlikely benefit of a mastectomy at all. Large, fixed tumours may be considered for preoperative neoadjuvant chemotherapy or hormonal therapy, to shrink the tumour mass and enable oncologically safer surgery with clear margins.

Procedure

The patient is **supine** under **general anaesthetic** with the ipsilateral arm **abducted** on an **arm board** at about 80 degrees. **Prep** and **drape** the whole of the breast up to well above the clavicle,

How to Operate: for MRCS Candidates and Surgical Trainees, First Edition. M. Stephenson. © 2011 John Wiley & Sons, Ltd. Published 2011 by John Wiley & Sons, Ltd.

well across the sternum and well below the inframammary fold. Prep into the axilla and the upper arm. Drape the breast, superiorly at the clavicle, medially just the other side of the sternum, inferiorly just below the inframammary fold and square it off laterally in the axilla (if continuing on to an axillary dissection, obviously keep all this undraped).

Marking the breast is important, you'll find those marks surprisingly helpful once you've started cutting and dissecting and everything looks distorted.

- The **medial edge** of the breast mound—the medial edge of dissection
- The **inframammary fold**—it can become unclear when stretched out and so helps when identifying the inferior limit of dissection
- The **superior edge** of the breast mound
- The **lateral edge** of breast tissue—often hanging down under the axilla
- The **midline**—so you don't ever accidentally excise beyond it (see later).

The next bit of marking is one of the most crucial bits of the operation and helps you work out how much skin to excise. It may sound long-winded but it will prevent the disaster of not having enough skin left to close up at the end, or too much.

Stand over the breast looking down, that is with an aerial view. Make a **horizontal mark** (**mark A**) on the **sternum** at the **level of the nipple**, and another mark (**mark B**) also at the level of the nipple, but at the **lateral edge** of the breast. Now hold onto the breast

with one hand and **pull it inferiorly**, fairly firmly. Draw a **straight line** right across the breast from mark A to B.

Next pull the breast mound **superiorly** and draw another straight line between mark A and B. Let go of the breast—hey presto, your two straight lines are magically converted into an **ellipse** around the nipple areolar complex. This will be the ellipse of skin to incise. Before you do that however, double-check that when you've excised that skin, the edges will **come comfortably together**. To do this, again simply stand looking down on the breast and fix your eyes on the line running between your mark A and B, let's call it the **horizon**. Pull the breast mound inferiorly then superiorly, and check that the two marked lines **overlap just slightly** at the horizon (holding your marker pen in the air horizontally over this horizon can help).

Now **incise** your skin ellipse going through **skin** and **superficial fascia** but no further. The superficial fascia is easily recognised and once you're through it you see the **fatty tissue** of the breast. The next step is to **raise** the **superior skin flap**. Using **skin hooks** or similar, ask your assistant to lift up the skin of the superior flap and start **dissecting** just under the skin. A plane is usually quite obvious, and you are separating the skin and underlying subcutaneous fat off from the mammary fat at the level of this superficial fascia. Take great care throughout not to make the flap too thin, risking buttonholing the skin, or too

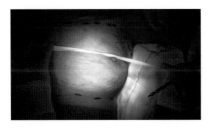

The tape of a large gauze swab is being used to guide where to make mark A and B. Note the dotted lines marking the edges of the breast tissue.

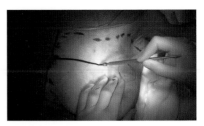

The breast is being pulled down and a line drawn between mark A and B.

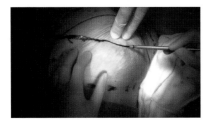

The breast is being pulled up.

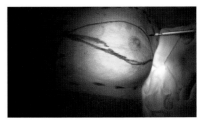

The skin ellipse.

thick leaving behind lumps of breast tissue.

So keep dissecting under the skin flap going right round the superior breast as far as your premarked **superior edge line**. You can use **bipolar diathermy scissors**, or **fingerswitch** diathermy or a simple, sharp scalpel with a big blade, for example a 22 blade. Some surgeons even prefer a pair of large curved non-diathermy scissors. Keep the usual monopolar diathermy forceps handy for haemostasis as you go along. Do this all the way round the upper half of the breast, paying particular attention to the **axillary tail**, which is an extension of breast tissue up into the axilla that needs to come too (leaving it results in an ugly lump and residual oncopotential tissue). Medially take care not to go beyond the premarked medial edge line—and definitely **not**

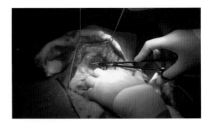

The superior skin flap is being lifted with skin hooks and a subfascial plane made with bipolar diathermy scissors.

beyond the midline. If you do this and the patient is going to have reconstructive surgery with implants, the implant might displace into the other side resulting in a deformity known as **synmastia**, where the juncture between breast and sternum is lost—very difficult to treat. Also medially take care for **branches of the internal mammary artery** that perforate through the pectoralis major—they can bleed and retract back into the muscle giving a painful postoperative chest wall haematoma, so stop them with diathermy before they do.

Once you've lifted the skin flap up in full, you need to dissect down deep onto **pectoralis fascia**. So you will have lifted the skin flap superiorly to just below the clavicle, and here turn your chosen instrument of dissection **perpendicular** to the chest wall and come down onto **pectoralis major**, which will be clearly seen through its covering fascia. Continue this all the way round the upper half of the breast. With inferior traction on the breast **dissect the breast mound off pectoralis fascia**, which is usually a very clearly

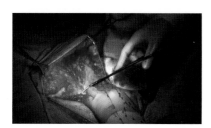

The breast is being retracted inferiorly and dissected off the pectoralis fascia.

seen plane, and the breast comes away pretty easily. Most people leave the pectoralis fascia *in situ*; this helps if reconstructing the breast as it holds the pectoralis muscle together, stopping it splitting.

Once you've dissected most of the breast off pectoralis fascia, **swap sides** with your assistant and repeat the process of flap dissection **inferiorly**. The plane here is usually slightly more unclear but the principles are the same. Again don't dissect further inferiorly than the **inframammary fold** mark. Doing so is not only unnecessarily traumatic but if the patient is to have reconstructive surgery, the recreated breast mound will **drop lower** than the other side. But conversely, don't leave any breast tissue here, this results in a **residual oncopotential ugly ridge**. See why the skin markings were so important?

Once the whole of the inferior skin flap is mobilised right round to the axilla, again turn your weapon **perpendicular** to the chest wall and get down to pectoralis fascia. All that remains is to continue dissecting the breast off the chest wall, which is usually best done by letting the weight of the breast hang down laterally and dissecting from medial to lateral with additional lateral traction on the breast. Make sure you don't leave any lumps of breast tissue behind.

Once the breast is clean off the chest wall, make sure you **mark it** for the pathologists. Laboratories vary in their practice but a good way is to put a stitch on the **superior** skin edge and cut it

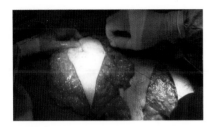

What the mastectomy specimen looks like. It's now being marked with stitches for the pathologists.

short and another stitch at the **lateral** skin edge and leave it **long** (**short = superior**, **long = lateral**), the nipple should hopefully give away where the anterior surface is.

Obviously if you need to also do an axillary procedure, now's the time to do it; often it's better to just continue the axillary dissection without completely removing the breast so that the breast specimen remains in continuity with the axillary sample. Next, make sure you've **stopped anything bleeding** by being meticulous with haemostasis on the chest wall and the skin flaps. **Wash out** the wound with, for instance, betadine flavoured water and then squirt some long-acting local anaesthetic into it. Insert a **suction drain** into the inferior part of the wound and

stitch it in with a non-absorbable suture. Now **close up;** techniques vary, but a cosmetically acceptable result comes from several **interrupted dermal stitches** followed by a **continuous subcutaneous** absorbable suture and steristrips. Cover with a **waterproof dressing**.

Notes

For bonus marks, you might like to know that there is the **skin-sparing mastectomy**—the same principles described here but a much smaller ellipse of skin is taken which can facilitate breast reconstruction. Lastly there's the **subcutaneous** or **nipple sparing mastectomy**, in which an incision in skin is made and the breast removed in the same way as described here, but no skin is actually excised. Generally this has only been in cases of **prophylactic mastectomies** for those at genetic high risk, but is likely to be less oncologically robust.

Occasionally, if the tumour is in a place far from the middle of the breast, say high in the upper outer quadrant and with skin involvement, you may need to adjust how you mark your skin ellipse, for instance shape it obliquely up to encompass the skin overlying the tumour.

Summary

- The patient is **supine**, under **general anaesthetic**, and the **arm abducted** to 80 degrees
- **Prep** and **drape** the breast
- **Mark** the medial, lateral, superior and inferior edges of the breast, and also the midline
- **Mark** the **skin ellipse**
- **Incise** the **skin ellipse**
- Raise the **superior skin flap**
- **Dissect** down to **pectoralis fascia** and begin **dissecting the breast off** the pectoralis fascia
- Raise the **inferior skin flap** and dissect down to pectoralis fascia
- Finish **dissecting the breast off** the pectoralis fascia, **mark it** and send to **histopathology**
- **Haemostasis, washout, suction drain** and **close**

31 Wide Local Excision

Matt Stephenson and Elizabeth F Shah

> **Video** | **9 min 56 s**
> Elizabeth F Shah, Consultant Oncoplastic Breast
> Surgeon, supervising Rudwan Adi
> Conquest Hospital, St Leonards-on-Sea

Introduction

Breast conserving surgery, that is removing the tumour without removing the whole of the breast, has increased in popularity over the years. Tumours that might otherwise have resulted in a mastectomy in the past are more likely to be managed with breast conserving surgery, which in the most part means a **wide local excision**—not a **lumpectomy** which is simply removing the lump—you want to remove the lump and the margin of macroscopically normal tissue around it.

But first, some points in general about where to make an **incision** on the breast, not just for wide locals. With both benign and malignant pathology, making a **cosmetically acceptable** scar is important.

- In general try to avoid the **upper part** of the breast unless absolutely necessary. Even with a lump in the superior part of the breast, you can make your skin incision lower and retract the skin edge up. These scars are highly visible, often don't heal quite so well and have a higher risk of keloid.
- Try to make your skin incision fit with the **curve of the breast** and ideally within the natural Langer's lines.
- When excising malignant tumours, you **don't need to excise** any skin, just make an incision over the lump and lift skin flaps. An exception to this is if the tumour is invading the overlying skin, in which case take an ellipse with the skin (like in this video as it happens).
- When excising fairly central lumps, a **periareolar scar** gives excellent access and cosmetic result.
- For breast implants, for instance in breast augmentation, an incision in the skin crease of the **inframammary fold** is very well hidden.

How to Operate: for MRCS Candidates and Surgical Trainees, First Edition. M. Stephenson. © 2011 John Wiley & Sons, Ltd. Published 2011 by John Wiley & Sons, Ltd.

- If you're doing a wide local excision, imagine where your **skin ellipse** would be if you were doing a mastectomy—if the margins are heavily involved, the patient may end up later having a **completion mastectomy**, and you'll want the wide local scar to be removed with the mastectomy, not be an additional one.
- If you're doing an incision and drainage of a lactational breast abscess, consider whether you could do repeat **needle aspirations**, say every day for a few days, and **antibiotics** rather than create a scar and risk a milk fistula.
- Closing the incision with **subcuticular absorbable suture** leaves no mark on the skin giving an excellent cosmetic result, and putting in a layer of **deep dermal** interrupted stitches takes the tension off the skin, reducing the risk of dehiscence.

Procedure

With the patient **supine**, **arm abducted** on an armboard and under **general anaesthetic**, **prep** and **drape** the whole of the breast. **Palpate** the lump and draw a **mark** around it to help you remember. Make an **incision** over the lump following the principles described above. You **don't** need to actually **excise** any skin unless you recognised obvious skin involvement such as **skin tethering** or **fixity** to skin during preoperative examination (you probably won't see this when the patient's asleep on the table). **Incise** through **skin**, **subcutaneous fat** and **superficial fascia**. Ask your assistant to **lift up** one flap with skin hooks or Allis forceps (on the subcutaneous surface not external skin) and **dissect** under the flap, so that you're just beyond the palpable lump which you keep hold of with your other hand. You can dissect with a knife, scissors or monopolar diathermy. Keep in the plane between subcutaneous fat and breast tissue.

Once you're beyond the lump by about a centimetre, turn your instrument **90 degrees** so it's **perpendicular** to the chest wall and dissect **straight down** to pectoralis major (or strictly speaking the thin fascia overlying it) keeping about **1 cm** of normal tissue between the growth and the dissection. Dissect straight down, go straight to pec major. Do not pass Go, do not collect £200, go straight down. This is crucial because an important oncological concept of wide local excision surgery is that you remove the

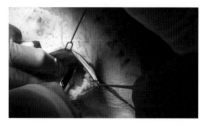

The surgeon's left hand is on the cancerous lump and the diathermy scissors in the right hand are dissecting under the skin flap, which is being elevated by skin hooks.

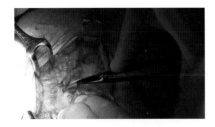

The skin flaps have been raised all around the tumour and the diathermy scissors are now pointing at 90 degrees to the chest wall coming straight down on to pectoralis fascia.

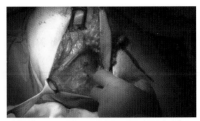

OK it doesn't much look like a cylinder here granted, but all the breast tissue has been resected from skin down to pectoralis fascia seen at the base of this wound (ordinarily it would be from just under the skin to pectoralis fascia).

cancer with a *cylinder* of tissue, stretching from just under the **skin flap** right down to the **pectoralis fascia**. There is a real risk of **undermining** the tumour or worse, cutting straight through it, if you don't do this. The main reason for abiding by this rule is that if the patient's deep or superficial margin is found to contain cancer, you will know that there will be no point in going back to theatre for re-excision as you will have already removed all the tissue in those directions—if it's invaded pectoralis or skin, there is no benefit in further local excision.

So far then you've made an incision, dissected one skin flap from over the lump and dissected straight down on to pectoralis keeping 1 cm of macroscopically normal tissue around the tumour. Now continue the dissection **circumferentially** around the tumour, again making sure that eventually what you remove will resemble a cylinder of tissue. Once you've dissected 180 degrees around the lump under the first skin flap you can actually start dissecting the whole cylinder **off**

the pectoralis fascia (even though you haven't done the other 180 degrees yet, you can still dissect off the bottom of the whole cylinder). Then **repeat** the same process for the other skin flap, if you've already dissected the whole of the cylinder base off the pectoralis you'll find you can easily deliver the developing cylinder out of the wound facilitating the remainder of the dissection. It is important at all times to keep in mind where the cancer is and ensure that you're keeping about **1 cm** of normal breast tissue around it—but **not too much** or you'll leave a large disfiguring cavity.

Once the cylinder is excised, **mark** it before you send it to the pathologists, for example by putting a **short** stitch **superiorly**, **long** stitch **laterally** and a **loop** of stitch **anteriorly**, or any other system previously agreed with your pathologists. Then, if one of the margins is involved, you will know which margin to re-excise when doing a cavity re-excision.

Take a Ligaclip and apply some **clips** to the margins of the breast cavity, halfway up between the pectoralis muscle and the skin, two superiorly, two medially, two laterally and two inferiorly. This will help guide the **radiotherapists** as to where to project their rays, as they undertake CT planning to guide radiotherapy treatment. In the olden days, the scar would be placed directly over the tumour bed but with the development of improved oncoplastic skills, the scar may have been placed in a more cosmetically acceptable place and dissection beneath a longer skin flap taken place, and therefore the scar may not indicate quite where the tumour was. It's also just more accurate anyway.

When closing, you don't need to close the cavity, this will just fill up with serous fluid and eventually organize into scar tissue. Just **close the skin** with deep dermal interrupted sutures and subcutaneous continuous absorbable suture to skin.

Notes

Whilst you're aiming for a 1-cm macroscopic margin, the minimum acceptable microscopic margin is **1 mm**. Less than this and the patient will need to return to theatre for **cavity re-excision**, that is open up the same scar and excise either the superior, inferior, medial or lateral margin by another centimetre depth or so (hence the importance of accurate marking). If there's still cancer present in this margin, they'll either need to have it done again, or thought given to a mastectomy. These decisions are made at breast multidisciplinary meetings.

The majority of cancers have come to light because the patient has noticed it themselves—it is therefore **palpable**. However **breast cancer screening** has brought another type of patient and problem—the cancer is **not palpable**, it's merely recognised as a shadow on a mammogram. In order to find these cancers therefore, they need to be radiologically identified preoperatively by ultrasound or mammography by inserting a **flexible wire** under local anaesthetic so that the tip is buried in the cancer. Your job is then to dissect out the tip of the wire—hoping that it hasn't moved position on the way from the radiology department to theatre, or that you don't cut through it during your dissection. This is the so called **wire-guided wide local excision**.

Summary

- The patient is **supine** with **arm abducted** under **general anaesthetic**
- The breast is **prepped** and **draped**
- **Mark** the lump
- **Choose** the incision
- **Incise** through **skin**, subcutaneous **fat** and **fascia**
- **Lift** one skin flap
- **Dissect** down to **pectoralis fascia**
- Complete **circumferentially**
- **Dissect off pec fascia**
- Lift the other skin flap and **repeat**
- Take out the **cylinder of tissue**
- **Mark** the cylinder
- **Clips** to pec fascia
- **Close** the skin

32 Axillary Node Clearance

Matt Stephenson and Elizabeth F Shah

> **Video** | **10 min 19 s**
> Elizabeth F Shah, Consultant Oncoplastic Breast Surgeon
> Conquest Hospital, St Leonards-on-Sea

Introduction

Many medical students don't have much exposure to breast surgery during their under-graduate years and then only sparsely as a doctor. It is therefore shrouded in mystery for many and never more so when it comes to the axilla. Which operation—sampling, clearance, sentinel node or nothing? Which patients need it? When to perform it, at the same time or later? What on earth is going on in that peculiar shaped, seemingly inaccessible tissue? Let's try to make it all perfectly clear.

A patient comes with a breast lump. She has **triple assessment**: a history and examination, radiological tests (usually ultrasound and mammography) and some form of pathological assessment (cytology or biopsy). It is found that she has a small cancerous growth in the lower pole of her breast. It is felt that this would be amenable to wide local excision followed by radiotherapy.

The wide local excision will deal (hopefully) with the local cancer but it will do nothing for her draining lymph nodes. You wouldn't be happy to excise someone's colonic cancer and not take the local lymph nodes in the mesentery would you? One of the most basic rules of oncological surgery is to take the **local draining lymph nodes**. Therefore, the gold standard has been to remove the axillary tissue containing those lymph nodes, at the same operation as for the lump. In the past, all the axillary tissue was taken, right up to level 3 up to the root of the neck. Research has shown however that going up to **level 2** (we'll come back to those levels later) alone is equally good in terms of onco-logical outcome with fewer cases of **lymphoedema**.

However, if you remove all those nodes on everyone with a breast cancer, the pro-portion of people actually having any positive lymph nodes is only about **25%**, so

How to Operate: for MRCS Candidates and Surgical Trainees, First Edition. M. Stephenson. © 2011 John Wiley & Sons, Ltd.
Published 2011 by John Wiley & Sons, Ltd.

three-quarters of them may have had it done unnecessarily. So **axillary node sampling** came into fashion—instead of removing all those axillary nodes, you still make an incision in the axilla as before but just carefully dissect the lower axilla (level 1, i.e. you don't need to retract pectoralis minor) actually looking for lymph nodes (which can be like looking for a needle in a haystack if they're tiny, and you have to resist the temptation to declare to the theatre in exasperation that you've found a lymph node when in fact you know perfectly well that it's a globule of fat—it'll come back to bite you in the Multi Disciplinary Meeting (MDM)). You take about four of them. In some hospitals, the operation would then end, and if at the MDM your lymph nodes are reported as having malignancy in them, the patient will need to come back to theatre another day to have a full clearance. In other hospitals they may have histopathological services on standby to rapidly assess your nodes whilst you're twiddling your thumbs in theatre, and if there's a malignancy there, you can proceed with the clearance at the same sitting.

A modification of this is **sentinel lymph node biopsy**. In this scenario, preoperatively a **radiocolloid solution** and/or intraoperatively **patent blue dye**, is injected intradermally into the breast. Both of these will rapidly (hours versus minutes, respectively) migrate through the lymphatics up into the axilla (you can watch the blue dye as it moves up). You can then hold a radioisotope detector over the skin of the axilla, and incise down over the 'hottest' patch, identify the node and dissect it out—hopefully it will also be blue. You may find multiple hot and/or blue nodes, that is most people have more than one sentinel node. Using both techniques increases the yield and stands in if the other technique doesn't work. In the same way as with the sampling, if the nodes are cancerous the patient needs a clearance—either at the same sitting or later.

Bear in mind that patients with **ductal carcinoma in situ** (DCIS) don't need any axillary surgery—this is a non-invasive growth and therefore shouldn't have metastasised to the axilla. However, patients with extensive DCIS needing mastectomy can be offered sentinel node biopsy of the axilla at the time of mastectomy.

Before we begin let's just remind ourselves of the **anatomy** of the axilla. It is a **pyramid- shaped** area of tissue in your armpit, the broad **square base** being the **skin** of the armpit and the **apex** being formed not quite at a point but of a small space with three borders: the **1st rib**, the **clavicle** and the **scapula**—but you're not going to get this deep to see it in your standard level 2 axillary clearance. The borders are:

Anteriorly: pectoralis minor and major (and a little bit of subclavius)
Posteriorly: subscapularis superiorly, teres major and latissimus dorsi inferiorly
Medially: the chest wall covered by serratus anterior
Laterally: the intertubercular sulcus of the humerus.

So what's with the levels? The pectoralis minor is a narrow, triangular, fairly weedy muscle compared to his brother pec major and crosses the front of the axilla obliquely from ribs 2, 3 and 4 up to the coracoid process of the scapula. It serves therefore as a useful marker of how deep into the axilla you are. Inferolateral to pec minor is level 1, directly behind pec minor is level 2 and superomedial to pec minor is level 3. The standard axillary clearance is level 2 or 3.

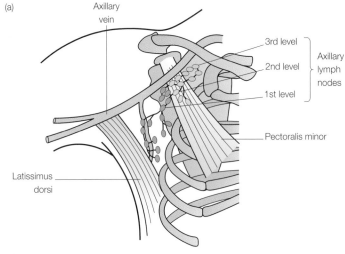

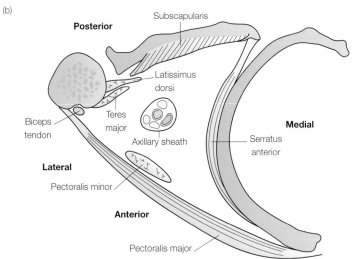

The axilla—its relations and contents.

Procedure

The patient is **supine** with the arm **abducted** at about 80 degrees. You may be approaching the axilla from one of two ways, either through a **separate incision** from a wide local excision which may be some way distant on the breast, or through the **same incision** as you've made for a mastectomy or an upper outer quadrant wide local excision.

In the case of the former, you need a **curved incision** running from back to front. **Palpate** the **latissimus dorsi**—the posterior border of the axilla, and the **pectoralis major**—the anterior border of the axilla. Your incision wants to run **between these**, but **not over them** which results in an ugly scar. How close to the armpit itself? In the lower axilla, a couple of fingerbreadths above where you can feel the rib cage disappearing off into the chest to be covered by fat.

In the case of the latter, the access is going to be much easier as you'll have a much larger wound to get to the axilla. When you've dissected the breast off the chest wall (see *Mastectomy* Chapter 30) at the lateral aspect you've already attained similar access to the above paragraph as you'll see from the video.

Either way, once you've made your incision you now want to actually see the muscles you just felt earlier on by palpation when you were deciding your site of incision. Get your assistant to **retract** the skin edges. The **first landmark** you want to identify is the **pectoralis major** and follow this down to its posterior edge,

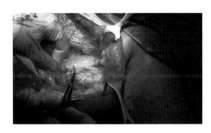

The axilla is being approached through the lateral end of the mastectomy wound. The surgeon's hand is feeling beneath the pec.

behind it you will find the pectoralis minor which your assistant will be able to retract up—these form the **anterior border** of the axilla. Next you want to identify the **posterior border**. So now go to the posterior limit of your wound and burrow down until you meet **latissimus dorsi** muscle. If you seem to be burrowing down too far, remember you may have gone too laterally and you're headed for the operating table instead. Once you've found it, everything in between is axilla. It's covered by **fascia** which you now need to **divide**, do this with diathermy. As soon as you've opened it, you see a different kind of fat—**axillary fat**, and this is quite obvious.

Use your non-dominant hand to **retract down** the axillary contents and with your assistant's retractor under the pectoralis major and minor, gradually **dissect** upwards underneath said pecs. As you dissect ever deeper, you may find a number of structures, including innominate veins and arteries but you will also find a stringy structure running

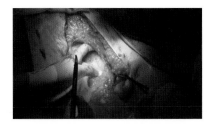

The edge of pec major can easily be seen. The fascia covering the axillary contents anteriorly is being divided.

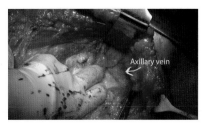

We've dissected through the axilla to find the axillary vein.

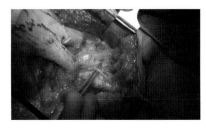

The intercostobrachial nerve is being demonstrated.

transversely through the axillary tissue—this is the **intercostobrachial nerve** running from chest wall to inner arm to supply sensation, there may be several branches. Often it's impossible to preserve these so you may need to cut them, at the medial edge and then again at the lateral edge, leaving the middle section within your specimen.

Now you're ready to find the **key to the axilla**—the **axillary vein**—the principal thing you don't want to damage but must keep in view ideally at all times the moment you enter the axilla, like some kind of worshipful deity to guide you but punish you for an incorrect manoeuvre.

Dissect deeper towards the **apex** of the axilla using a combination of sharp dissection with scissors and blunt dissection, say with a **pledget**. Looking always, for *big blue*—the axillary vein—running across the posterior wall of the axilla from neck to arm. When you see it, you've reached the upper limit of how far in you need to go. Gently **dissect the tissue off the vein** (taking great care not to damage it) so that the specimen starts to **peel off** the posterior wall.

So far then you've begun the dissection of the anterior and posterior borders and figured out how far in you'll need to go. Next you need to start on the **medial** and **lateral** walls. **Serratus anterior** will come into view and you'll see it's covering the rib cage. Following on from identifying the crucial structure of the axillary vein you're looking for the next important structure: the **long thoracic nerve of Bell**. It's running **vertically** down the **medial side** of the chest wall on serratus anterior just behind the mid axillary line. Preserve it! It's supplying serratus anterior and if you damage it

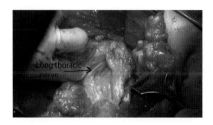

The long thoracic nerve is glimpsed running down the chest wall on serratus anterior.

the patient ends up with the ugly deformity of **winging of the scapula**. Gently dissect the axillary contents off it.

The next important structure to identify and preserve is the **thoracodorsal pedicle**. This is a bundle of artery, vein and nerve descending from the axillary artery, vein and brachial plexus respectively, but by the time they've all met up at the level of the axillary vein, they like to stay close to each other. They supply the latissimus dorsi. The main reason they're important is if you are going to proceed to **latissimus dorsi flap** reconstruction of the breast. You'll find it by dissecting inferiorly to the axillary vein along the

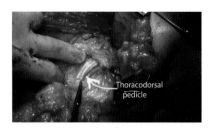

The thoracodorsal pedicle is seen running down the front of latissimus dorsi.

posterior wall of the axilla. You need to keep it on the posterior wall of the axilla (i.e. the lat dorsi) and not let it pull up with the axillary contents which it often has a mind to do. Sometimes it has an anterior branch entering the axilla which you can ligate and divide.

Once you've identified the axillary vein as your principle landmark, begun dissection down the medial, posterior and lateral walls and identified and preserved those two important structures, the rest is plain sailing. Get **Allis forceps** on the axillary tissue and retract it down out of the wound to help with the dissection. If you can take the whole pyramid of tissue out in one block, all the better, but often (and especially if you've tried to preserve the intercostobrachial nerve as we did in our video) it needs to come out in fragments. Once you've taken out the bulk of the specimen, it's crucial to **review each border** to look for remaining axillary tissue that could be harbouring nodes. Removing the axillary tissue up to the axillary vein is roughly all the tissue behind pec minor (which has been retracted) and so is called a level 2 clearance. However, you should now **feel** with your fingers deep in the axilla, around and above the axillary vein and beyond pectoralis minor, as well as in the groove between pec major and minor, to check for obvious remaining pathological feeling nodes which would need to be extracted piecemeal. Make sure you put a **short stitch** in the axillary specimen at the **apex** of the dissection to help the pathologist identify the **apical**

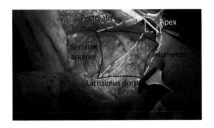

The axilla has been emptied. The borders are labelled in black and the white lines show the axilla projected up into the apex in the neck.

node, or if removed separately, put it in a separate pot.

The axillary wound tends to **ooze** a lot of serous fluid which isn't surprising given all that lymphatic tissue you've just cut through, **postoperative seromas** are very common. Ensure **haemostasis**. Insert a **suction drain** into the axilla to drain the worst of any early postoperative ooze and secure it in place with a non-absorbable stitch. **Close** the wound with **interrupted dermal stitches** and then a continuous absorbable **subcutaneous** stitch for the skin. Cover with a **water-proof dressing**.

Summary

- Make a **curved incision** in the axilla or continue from the **lateral edge** of the mastectomy wound
- **Dissect** down and identify **pectoralis major**
- **Dissect** down and identify **latissimus dorsi**
- **Dissect** into the axilla
- Ligate or preserve **intercostobrachial nerve**
- Identify the **axillary vein**
- Begin **dissecting out the block** of axillary contents from the medial, posterior and lateral walls
- Identify and preserve the **long thoracic nerve**
- Identify and preserve the **thoracodorsal pedicle**
- Remove any **remnants** of axillary tissue
- **Palpate** into level 3 for obviously pathological nodes
- Ensure **haemostasis**, insert **drain** and **close**

33 Fibroadenoma

Matt Stephenson and Elizabeth F Shah

> **Video** | **2 min 58 s**
> Elizabeth F Shah, Consultant Oncoplastic Breast Surgeon
> Conquest Hospital, St Leonards-on-Sea

Introduction

Breast surgery's not all about cancer you know. Thankfully you'll diagnose a lot **more benign** breast lumps in clinic than malignant ones. If triple assessment of the lump is reassuring, most of these lumps can be **left alone**. Some of them, however, will still arouse suspicion even if just in the patient, and are best removed.

Benign **cysts** of course can just be **aspirated** with a needle and syringe without local anaesthetic in the clinic, however solid lumps will require excision in theatre. Generally, breast lumps will require a general anaesthetic as getting good anaesthesia is difficult with local infiltration, especially if deep. Skin lesions on the breast, however, are usually amenable to local anaesthetic like elsewhere on the body.

The commonest benign lump is the **fibroadenoma** although you can find a lipoma in the breast or some women have particularly nodular breast tissue giving the impression of lumps—excision here is certainly not indicated and can be more tricky to manage. Fibroadenomas are typically in **younger** women, highly **mobile** and **smooth**.

This is a **lumpectomy**—different from a wide local excision—you are just trying to remove the lump, not a margin of macroscopically normal cylinder of tissue. Minimise the amount of normal breast tissue you remove.

Procedure

The lump should previously have been located and marked out on the surface of the breast, with the patient awake. With the patient **supine**, arm **abducted** and under **general anaesthetic**, **prep** and **drape** the breast. Now decide on your incision—follow the principles of good breast incisions in the *Wide Local Excision* introduction, Chapter 31.

Incise through **skin**, **subcutaneous fat** down onto the lump, which is kept

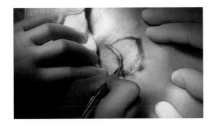

The left hand is over the nipple and the right hand is incising the blue mark, which has been drawn around the areola—a periareolar incision. The black mark indicates the location of the lump.

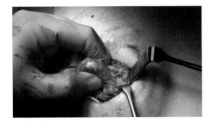

The left hand is holding the fibroadenoma, pulling it out of the wound. The upper skin flap is being retracted with Langenbeck retractors; you can clearly see where the plane of dissection needs to be.

controlled by your non-dominant hand as these lumps can be very mobile. Here you don't have to raise skin flaps as you don't need a cylinder of tissue. **Retracting** the skin edge up with skin hooks or similar to give you space to operate, however, is essential. Dissect **straight down** to the lump and then **dissect round it**, again using your non-dominant hand to control it. Once you get round the back of the lump, **undermine it** and try to **flip it out** of the wound; this will make the rest of the dissection even easier. If the lump is very slippery and difficult to control, take a clip and grasp just the tissue immediately attached to the lump to help manipulate it. Dissect all the way round keeping close to the lump and eventually **deliver** it and **send** it for histopathological assessment. You don't need to mark it.

Establish **haemostasis** in the tissues and just **close the skin** (not the cavity, this will fill with serous fluid which will later organise) with **deep dermal** sutures and a continuous **subcutaneous absorbable** suture.

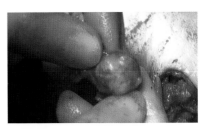

The fibroadenoma specimen.

Summary

- The patient is **supine** with **arm abducted** under **general anaesthetic**
- **Prep** and **drape** the breast
- Make a **cosmetically suitable** incision
- **Incise** through skin, subcutaneous fat and down almost onto the lump
- **Retract** the skin edges
- **Dissect** around the lump **keeping close** to it
- **Undermine** it and deliver it out of the wound
- Complete the **dissection**
- **Send** to the histopathologists
- **Close** the skin

34 Thyroidectomy

Matt Stephenson and John S Weighill

> **Video** | **9 min 9 s**
> John S Weighill, Consultant ENT/Head and Neck
> Surgeon
> Royal Sussex County Hospital, Brighton

Introduction

Once a standard general surgical operation, you're now much more likely to only come across this one in an ENT job. If it weren't for the fact that there are some rather important structures in this area, like laryngeal nerves, the trachea, the common carotid artery and the parathyroids, it would be an easy operation . . . Nevertheless if you know the anatomy well, you should be able to avoid disaster.

Procedure

With the patient in the **reverse Trendelenburg position** (head of bed raised to **empty the veins** in the neck) and under **general anaesthetic**, with the help of the anaesthetist **extend the neck**. This will open up the anterior neck and also may help lift a large retrosternal thyroid out from the mediastinum. This is accomplished by a pillow or similar **under the shoulders** and **supporting the head** in a head ring. In the elderly, with arthritic necks it may not be possible to extend the neck much. **Prep** and **drape** the neck wrapping the head in a separate head drape.

So now you need to choose where you will make your skin incision. This is a **curved incision** within the skin crease at a level **halfway** between the **cricoid** and the **suprasternal notch**, which you can easily palpate. **Infiltrate** along your planned incision with lignocaine mixed with adrenaline. Now make your incision. It should be a **curved incision**, don't let it drift too transversely and end up going over the clavicles which gives an

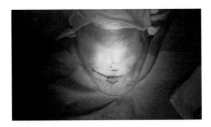

The cricoid is marked superiorly and suprasternal notch inferiorly, the curvilinear line in between is the line of incision.

How to Operate: for MRCS Candidates and Surgical Trainees, First Edition. M. Stephenson. © 2011 John Wiley & Sons, Ltd. Published 2011 by John Wiley & Sons, Ltd.

ugly scar. You can cut straight through **skin**, **superficial fascia** and **platysma**. Beneath this is the **investing layer of deep fascia** (the most superficial layer of fascia that's continuous all the way round the neck enveloping some of the muscles), and you want to **create a plane** just superficial to this.

So take the **upper edge** of the wound with tissue forceps and **dissect underneath** the **platysma**, over the deep fascia. Now do this for the **lower edge**. You can hold these two edges apart with a rather elegant retractor, the **Joll retractor**. If you look now at the base of the wound, it's covered with deep fascia. To get through this plane find the **midline**, make an incision and then **cut up** and **down** with some dissecting scissors. This is right in between the **strap muscles** of the neck, the **sternothyroid** and **sternohyoid**, so if you stick to the midline it's fairly bloodless.

Once you're through, lift up the strap muscles overlying whichever half of the gland you're after with the aid of a **Langenbeck retractor**. You now need to

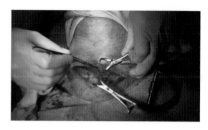

Joll retractors to retract the skin edges.

peel off the strap muscles from the underlying gland by a combination of **sharp** and **blunt dissection**. As you get round the lateral edge of the gland you need to start thinking about the arteries and veins going into or out of the gland. Firstly, there's the **middle thyroid vein** (no middle thyroid artery remember) which may or may not be present. **Ligating** and **dividing** this **early** will help with **mobilising** the thyroid, that is lifting it out of the neck into the wound so it's easier to see around it. Work your way around the gland **superiorly** keeping close to the gland. Next, you're looking for the superior thyroid vein and artery, which may be very close together.

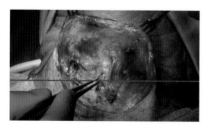

The superior skin edge has being retracted and made into a flap exposing the investing fascia of the neck.

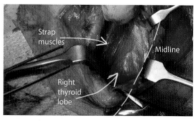

The right thyroid lobe is exposed by retracting the strap muscles.

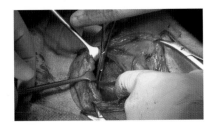

The Langenbecks are still retracting the strap muscles laterally, the thyroid is being pulled medially and the middle thyroid vein has been clipped.

Rather unfortunately for us all, the thyroid is **irritatingly close** to the larynx and that means that two of the nerves heading for the larynx to supply the muscles of speech cross the territory of your thyroidectomy. Now you have to actually be able to **understand** the anatomy of the nerves in this region and not just be able to recite Last's anatomy *ad verbatim*. At the top of the gland

there's a nerve to be wary of and another one at the inferior end. **Superiorly**, it's the **external laryngeal nerve. Inferiorly**, it's the **recurrent laryngeal nerve**.

Let's start at the **top**. The **external laryngeal nerve** is the smaller of the two branches of the **superior laryngeal nerve** (which is a branch of the **vagus** nerve) which descends beside the pharynx. The external laryngeal nerve continues its descent close to and **deep to the superior thyroid artery** (which has branched and descended from the external carotid artery from above) and supplies the **cricothyroid** muscle, which helps to **tense** the vocal cords. Damage to it results in a **hoarse voice**. If you were to ligate the superior thyroid artery you would therefore want to do so **after** the nerve has entered the cricopharyngeus. So it makes sense to **ligate the artery as close to the gland as you can**, after

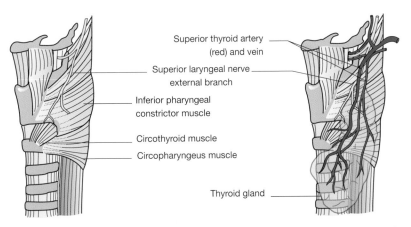

Superior thyroid artery (red) and vein

Superior laryngeal nerve external branch

Inferior pharyngeal constrictor muscle

Circothyroid muscle

Circopharyngeus muscle

Thyroid gland

On the left is the external laryngeal nerve alone and on the right is the relationship with the superior thyroid artery.

it's said goodbye to its companion the external laryngeal nerve.

The **recurrent laryngeal nerve** supplies the **motor function** to the larynx, damage to it can result in a **hoarse voice**—not usually immediately but after a few weeks when the vocal cord has had a chance to atrophy. There is also the risk of **dysphagia** and **aspiration**, and with **bilateral** recurrent laryngeal nerve injury—**airway obstruction** ranging from mild stridor to complete obstruction.

The recurrent laryngeal nerve has a different course on each side, being **double** **the length** on the left and hence **more at risk** from other non-thyroidectomy injuries or pathology. On the **right**, the recurrent laryngeal nerve **descends** from the vagus nerve in the neck and **hooks** around the **subclavian artery** descending on the front of it and re-ascending posteriorly. On the **left** it's descending **even further** to hook around the **ligamentum arteriosum** below the aortic arch to hook back up into the neck again. On each side it's aiming for the **groove** between the **trachea** and the **oesophagus** so that it can enter the larynx. If it

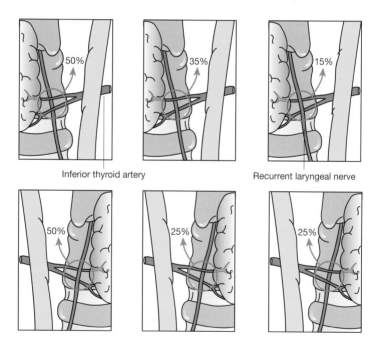

Inferior thyroid artery   Recurrent laryngeal nerve

The relationship of the recurrent laryngeal nerve (going roughly vertically) to the inferior thyroid artery (going roughly transversely), above show the left side, below is the right. It's demonstrating the variability in how the terminal branches of the inferior thyroid artery crosses the nerve.

were already in the groove at the level of the thyroid, like the books often suggest, then you'd have little to worry about as it would be consistent and easy to avoid, however this isn't the case. It is slightly more likely on the left however, as you might imagine as it's had more time to get there (that's the only direct relevance of the different recurrent courses to this operation—it means that injury on the right is more likely in thyroidectomy because it has a more oblique course—but left recurrent laryngeal palsy is more likely overall if you take into account other pathology such as mediastinal malignancy). Imagine then that you have reflected medially the thyroid lobe and you're looking at the bed from whence it lay. Coursing along the bed **obliquely** you may find the nerve going from **inferolateral** to **superomedial**, or it may already be very medial.

Almost at **right angles** to this nerve comes the **inferior thyroid artery**, a branch of the thyrocervical trunk (see the figure below showing the relationship of the recurrent laryngeal nerve to the inferior thyroid artery). On each side the relationship of the artery to the nerve varies in terms of whether the artery is **anterior**, **posterior** or **splits** around it, but in any event, the closer to the gland you get, the **friendlier** the artery and nerve have become. Regardless of all this therefore, the **further lateral** you ligate the inferior thyroid artery, the **less likely** you are to **prang the nerve**. Alternatively some surgeons prefer to meticulously expose all of

the nerve and divide all the little branches individually close to the gland and it's if you're doing the latter that the variability in their relationship becomes more relevant.

Also on the bed where the thyroid lobe lay are the **parathyroid glands**, usually two on each side. They may range from the size of a grain of rice to the size of a pea. Take care to avoid them if you see them. If you're doing a total thyroidectomy, it's much more important to identify at least one of them to make sure you're not either accidentally removing them or ruining their blood supply. They take their blood from the inferior thyroid artery so if you're going to stick to the rule of ligating the inferior thyroid artery far from the gland, you may **devascularise** them all leading to postoperative **severe hypocalcaemia**. If you're doing a total thyroidectomy therefore you will need to ensure that at least one of the parathyroids still has its blood supply.

When diathermying close to the nerves only use **bipolar diathermy**, not monopolar to reduce the extent of collateral tissue damage. **Ligate** all the vessels **well**—a postoperative bleed in a small

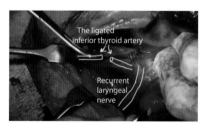

The inferior thyroid artery has been cut laterally.

space like the neck can compress the airway and be life threatening. Keep retracting the **thyroid medially** with your swabbed finger. Once you've divided those vessels it will become very mobile, all that will remain is to **detach** it from the **isthmus** of the thyroid and the **ligament of Berry** (which attaches it to the trachea). You can get a clip around these and ligate them. Bear in mind that the recurrent laryngeal nerve often tries to get in on the action here, being pulled up along with the retracted thyroid—take great care that it's staying put and not coming with the specimen. Obviously if you're doing a total or subtotal thyroidectomy, you need carry on and do pretty much the same thing on the other side.

Make a final check on **haemostasis**—be **meticulous**. If in doubt put in a **suction drain** that you can remove the next day. When closing, don't close the strap muscles together—that way if there is a postoperative bleed, the blood can leak out and be released by simply opening the skin. Just **close the platysma** and **skin** therefore. If you're concerned about bleeders that you may have missed, you can ask the anaesthetist to perform an **anaesthetic Valsalva** manoeuvre which raises the pressure in the veins in the neck and will identify any potential bleeding points before closing. Apply **Steristrips** and a **waterproof dressing**.

Summary

- The patient is in the **reverse Trendelenburg position** with the **neck extended** and head on a **head ring**
- **Prep** and **drape** the neck
- Make **curved incision** in the neck
- Raise superior and inferior **skin flaps**
- Dissect through the **midline**
- **Retract the strap muscles** of the neck laterally
- **Dissect** the thyroid lobe **drawing it medially**
- Ligate the **middle thyroid vein**
- Ligate the **superior thyroid vessels close** to the gland
- **Identify** the recurrent laryngeal nerve
- Ligate the **inferior thyroid artery away** from the gland
- Complete the **dissection**
- Ligate the **ligament of Berry** and the **isthmus** and send for histology
- Ensure **haemostasis** and consider a **drain**
- **Close** the platysma and **skin**

35 Tracheostomy

Matt Stephenson and John S Weighill

> **Video** | **10 min 28 s**
> John S Weighill, Consultant ENT/Head and Neck
> Surgeon
> Royal Sussex County Hospital, Brighton

Introduction

Time was, tracheostomies kept general and ENT surgeons pretty busy. These days however the majority of tracheostomies are done **percutaneously** (the percutaneous dilatational tracheostomy) on ITU by the anaesthetists. It's still a key skill to have however, especially in that most urgent of emergencies—actual or impending upper airway obstruction. One of the commonest scenarios for a formal surgical tracheostomy is as a precursor to head and neck surgery in which the upper airway is to be radically altered, for instance by a laryngectomy.

Procedure

The patient is in the **reverse Trendelenburg** position (head up to empty the neck veins), with a pillow behind the shoulders and the head supported in a **head ring**—this **extends** the cervical

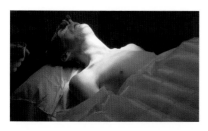

The neck is extended by putting a pillow beneath the shoulders and placing the head in a head ring.

spine, and thus **opens up** the front of the neck. The patient is usually under **general anaesthetic** but it can be done under local. **Prep** and **drape** the neck.

The incision is at the same level as for a thyroidectomy. Find the **suprasternal notch** and the **cricoid cartilage**—you need to make a **transverse incision** halfway between these two. It doesn't need to be as long as that for a thyroidectomy however—just a short horizontal incision. Even if the patient is under anaesthetic, infiltration with **local anaesthetic** before incising is sensible. In the event of a true emergency, you can make a **vertical** incision. Since the remainder of the

How to Operate: for MRCS Candidates and Surgical Trainees, First Edition. M. Stephenson. © 2011 John Wiley & Sons, Ltd.
Published 2011 by John Wiley & Sons, Ltd.

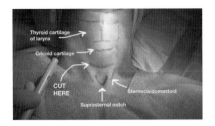

The landmarks have been marked and labelled.

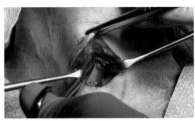

These Langenbecks retract the strap muscles laterally and the scissors dissect in the midline.

dissection continues in this direction it makes it slightly quicker at the expense of cosmesis—but who cares about that as long as the patient is alive.

Make your transverse incision through the **skin** and **subcutaneous fat**, through **platysma** and you'll find yourself in a fascial plane. There are **strap muscles** (so called because they're long thin rectangular structures) running **vertically** each side of the midline. There are **three layers** of them from outside to inside: **sternohyoid**, **sternothyroid with thyrohyoid** and, lastly, **omohyoid**. You want to enter the **midline** between them, which should be a relatively **avascular** plane. Ask your assistant to retract the strap muscles each side with **Langenbeck retractors** or similar and use scissors to **dissect down in the midline**. Obtain **haemostasis** as you go. If you do come across the **thyroid isthmus**, retract it **superiorly**.

You'll soon come down on to the **trachea** (feel it on yourself—it's not very deep). **Dissect around this**, opening up a pretracheal space. You'll then see the

white rings of the trachea—the aim is for your tracheostomy to be between the **third and fourth rings** down from the cricoid, so feel with your fingers up to the cricoid and count down the rings.

Before proceeding any further, **check your tracheostomy tube**. A man needs on average an **8 French**, versus a **6 to 7 French** for a woman. There should be an **outer tube** and a separate **inner tube** that slides into the outer tube—the purpose of that is that it can be removed intermittently and cleaned. There should also be an **introducer** with a blunt end that slots into the outer tube. Also check that you can **inflate the cuff**. You don't

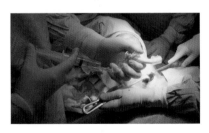

The cuff of the tracheostomy is being tested by insufflation.

want to find the inner component doesn't fit the outer component or that the cuff has a puncture after the anaesthetist has withdrawn their definitive airway.

You're now ready to **open the trachea** and put the tracheostomy in. This is when **coordination with the anaesthetist is crucial**. They need to be ready to remove their endotracheal tube when you're ready to insert your tracheostomy.

For a **non-permanent tracheostomy**—make a **horizontal slit** between the rings. For a **permanent tracheostomy**—you should **excise a thin ellipse** of tracheal wall. In **children**, a **vertical slit** should be made to minimise the risk of late tracheal stenosis. Let the anaesthetist know you're about to open the trachea and they can start withdrawing their endotracheal tube. As soon as you've opened the trachea, you'll hear **air escaping**. Use tracheal dilators to open up the hole and hold it open to insert the tube. It's usually easier to insert it so it seems to be pointing **superiorly at first** and then gently **rotating** it when the tip is inside. **Replace** the introducer with the inner tube.

Once it's in position, **reconnect** the anaesthetic tubing. Looking at the **expired CO_2** trace on the anaesthetic monitor will help confirm it's in the right place. **Inflate** the cuff.

All that remains is to **stitch** the tracheostomy in place—there are small holes in the sides of the tracheostomy to suture to. These don't need to be tight—a little movement to allow for the fact that the patient will move his head postoperatively is fine. **Taping** it to neck is also sensible. As long as you haven't made the incision too big, the skin doesn't need closing around the stoma.

Notes

People often confuse a **cricothyroidostomy** with a tracheostomy. A cricothyroidostomy is an emergency procedure to be performed in dire emergencies where there is sudden loss of a patent airway, for instance in upper airway trauma or severe burns. It is best known through the Advanced Trauma Life Support course.

If you're in this unfortunate scenario, you need to act **very fast**. You don't have

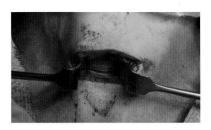

A horizontal tracheotomy has been made between the third and fourth tracheal rings.

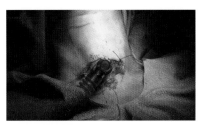

The finished product secured by stitches.

time to call an ENT surgeon or get out a tracheostomy set in A and E. The first time you'll do one, you'll never have seen one before. That doesn't mean you shouldn't do it if there is no other way of obtaining a definitive airway. Feel for the cricoid cartilage and feel the groove just above this before you come onto the thyroid cartilage of the larynx. Take a blade and make a horizontal stab incision in that groove right through the front of the trachea. Turn the blade around to use the handle and twist it around in the hole you just made (by this point the patient will have been anesthetised or have become so obtunded to be unaware of your actions). Insert the cricothyroidostomy tube and connect the anaesthetic tubing. It will need to be converted to a formal tracheostomy once the patient's condition allows.

It's also possible to just insert an intravenous cannula through the cricothyroid membrane and insufflate oxygen through this. It doesn't buy you a lot of time as it's an insufficient system to also blow off CO_2.

Summary

- The patient is under **general anaesthetic** in the **reverse Trendelenburg** position
- **Extend the neck**, **prep** and **drape**
- **Incise transversely**, halfway between cricoid and suprasternal notch
- Incise through **skin**, **subcutaneous fat** and **platysma**
- **Dissect in the midline**
- **Expose** the **trachea**
- **Check** the components of the **tracheostomy tube**
- In coordination with the anaesthetist, **incise the trachea**
- **Open the tracheotomy** with dilators and insert the tracheostomy tube
- **Check position**
- **Secure** in place

36 Haemorrhoidectomy

Matt Stephenson and Peter J Webb

> **Video** | **11 min 43 s**
> Peter J Webb, Consultant General and Colorectal
> Surgeon
> Medway Maritime Hospital, Gillingham

Introduction

In order to help maintain faecal continence, humans have some soft, squishy, blood-vessel-filled pads lining the anus. They're in the roughly **3, 7 and 11 o'clock** positions were you to inspect the anus head on with the patient lying on his back, legs spread, and draw the hours of the clock around it. Ordinarily they'd be helpful to us, but if they become enlarged, through **chronic straining** (resulting in that pad becoming engorged due to the Valsalva manoeuvre) to **pass a hard stool** (which drags down the mucosa of said engorged pad), they become an absolute nuisance and become known as **haemorrhoids**, or **piles**.

Firstly, being vascular structures, they tend to **bleed**. Usually being of the streaks of bright red blood on the toilet paper variety, or dripping into the toilet bowl. **Secondly**, they can bulge and be an **uncomfortable lump** that pokes out of the anus. **Thirdly**, they can acutely **thrombose** and bulge out of the anus, which is extremely painful. **Fourthly**, they can cause **perianal symptoms**, such as **itching** and difficulties maintaining perianal hygiene, since they disrupt the natural continence mechanism they're supposed to be there for.

Haemorrhoids can be classified according to the degree to which they prolapse, and this helps you decide how to treat them.

1st degree: can only be inspected on proctoscopy, it doesn't prolapse out

2nd degree: prolapses out of the anus but spontaneously reduces

3rd degree: prolapses out and requires digital reduction by the patient

4th degree: can't be reduced.

Management options include **conservative measures**, as a minimum for all, such as **increasing dietary fibre** intake, drinking **more water** (it's no good eating loads of fibre if the fibre isn't well hydrated in the colon to give it a bulking effect) and if necessary

How to Operate: for MRCS Candidates and Surgical Trainees, First Edition. M. Stephenson. © 2011 John Wiley & Sons, Ltd.
Published 2011 by John Wiley & Sons, Ltd.

laxatives. For **1st and 2nd degree** haemorrhoids, the mainstay of treatment is either **banding** or **injection** of oily phenol, both are usually done in outpatients. The former involves inspecting the internal extent of the haemorrhoid on proctoscopy, applying suction to the mucosa at the base of the haemorrhoid which raises it up like a bleb, and then applying a small rubber band to this, therefore constricting the blood flow to the haemorrhoid. The latter involves a similar approach but instead of the band, oily phenol is injected into the base of the pile causing it to shrivel up. Understandably, these don't show very well on video.

For symptomatic **3rd and 4th degree** haemorrhoids, banding or injections won't work so these patients require formal **haemorrhoidectomy**—excision of the haemorrhoids. The standard is the **Milligan–Morgan haemorrhoidectomy**. It has the benefit of essentially curing the patient of his haemorrhoids, but with the disadvantage of being extremely painful in the first week or two postoperatively. These patients need a significant amount of **laxatives** to keep the stool soft to pass postoperatively, **non-steroidal anti-inflammatories** and, often, **opiate** drugs (with extra laxatives to counter the side effects of these). Oral **metronidazole** postoperatively can also reduce postoperative pain.

Newer techniques have also been developed including the **stapled haemorrhoidectomy** and Doppler-guided transanal **haemorrhoidal artery ligation (HAL)**.

Procedure

The patient is under **general anaesthetic** and in the **lithotomy** position, with the **head down**, to help reduce venous engorgement of the haemorrhoids and to make them more at eye level. **Prep** and **drape** the anus and perianal area, ensuring that in a man, the scrotum is held out of the way (often the best way to do this is to simply use the patients own hand). Sterility is somewhat relative in an operation on the anus.

Sit down on a stool facing the anus, and once you're sitting comfortably, you may begin. Perform an **examination of the anus** and **perianal area** for other pathology including a digital rectal examination. Insert an **Eisenhammer retractor** into the anus and **examine circumferentially** the anal lining and identify the haemorrhoidal cushions that you're there to sort out. Sometimes you find only one offending haemorrhoid and the other two are inconsequential and can be left

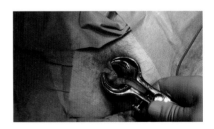

An Eisenhammer has been inserted—a prolapsing haemorrhoid is seen in the roughly 11 o'clock position.

alone, or just banded or injected. Usually, all three need excision and leaving a moderately enlarged one is tempting fate—you'll probably have to go back at a later date to excise that one too (in the video, this patient has already had one haemorrhoid excised elsewhere and has now come for the other two).

Use a **clip**, such as a **Spencer–Wells artery forceps** to clip the **mucocutaneous junction** of the haemorrhoid and use this to draw it out of the anus and then place **another clip** on it further **proximally**. You can use a further clip and pass this through the handles of the first two clips and clip it onto the drape, thus effectively keeping it, and the clips, out of the way. **Repeat** this for all the haemorrhoids.

Haemorrhoids are full of blood and thus tend to bleed a lot when operated on, so **inject some local anaesthetic**— such as **bupivacaine** with **1 : 200 000 adrenaline**—directly into the haemorrhoidal cushion and also the mucocutaneous junction, with the duel benefits of reducing pain and vasoconstricting.

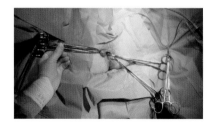

The haemorrhoids have been retracted outwards and their clips held with an additional clip.

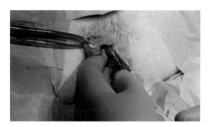

Injection of lignocaine with adrenaline.

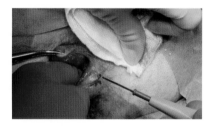

Skin incision.

Using the **diathermy finger switch** (although this was traditionally done with scissors) **excise the skin** around the haemorrhoid, sticking close to the mucocutaneous junction. Start with the haemorrhoid that's lowermost, otherwise if you do the uppermost one first, by the time you get to the lower one, you'll have a constant drip of blood from the first one on to your operative field, which is irritating.

Retraction by your assistant is crucial in this operation—they need to retract the perianal skin away from the anus and help to regularly dab the wound with a swab, whilst you retract the haemorrhoid in the opposite direction by a combination of traction on the clips and pinching

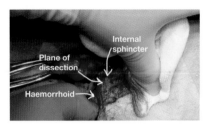

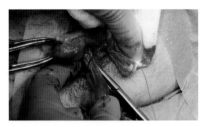

The haemorrhoid is being peeled off the internal sphincter. Note the counter traction between assistant and operator.

Transfixion of the haemorrhoidal base.

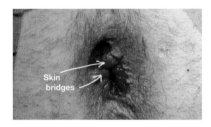

Bridges of skin are retained between the wounds (only two haemorrhoids have been excised here).

the haemorrhoid between finger and thumb. This will help to **open up a plane** between the haemorrhoid and the underlying tissue, primarily—the **internal sphincter**—which is an easily palpable ring of firm tissue around the anal canal, and is white in colour. The haemorrhoid is like a slug that's wrapped itself around the internal sphincter, and your task is to peel it off with the diathermy. You do not want to include the internal sphincter in your excision!

Continue the dissection until the haemorrhoid is attached only by a narrow base of tissue and **transfix** this firmly with a strong absorbable tie such as 0 Vicryl—leave this long—don't cut it yet, but you can now **cut off the haemorrhoid** with a pair of scissors. Repeat this for the other haemorrhoids. Crucially, you **must leave a bridge of skin** between each wound or else the patient is at risk of **anal stenosis** when the wounds heal and scar up.

You're now left with the transfixion stitch threads hanging out of the anus from each of the haemorrhoids. Reposition the Eisenhammer and **inspect**

the wound bases and **check for bleeding**—be quite meticulous with the haemostasis stage. Having the transfixion stitch threads still on the haemorrhoid bases helps to locate them and gently coax them down (without pulling them off) to check they're not bleeding.

Once you're happy with the haemostasis, insert a **haemostatic pack** (greased with some lubricating jelly) like a Spongostan into the anus and use some **non-adherent dressings** like Jelonet to cover the wounds, over which you can place some **sterile surgical pads**. Obviously the haemostatic pack doesn't stay in for long, it's really just there for the first few hours after the operation when the patient may cough on waking from the anaesthetic which may cause more oozing. It should pass naturally (in fact it's often fallen out by the time the patient's back on the ward) before the patient goes home. It's generally advised that for a few days before and after the operation the patient takes some **laxatives** so the stool is easier to pass.

Summary

- The patient is under **general anaesthetic** in the **lithotomy position** with the **head down**
- **Prep** and **drape** the anus and perianal area
- **Examine the anus** and perianal area carefully
- **Put a clip** on the mucocutaneous junction and body of each haemorrhoid
- **Inject** with **bupivocaine** mixed with 1 : 200 000 **adrenaline**
- **Excise** the **skin** around the haemorrhoid with diathermy
- **Deepen the dissection** peeling the haemorrhoid off the internal sphincter
- **Transfix** the base of the haemorrhoid
- **Repeat** for other haemorrhoids maintaining skin bridges
- Ensure **haemostasis**
- Insert **haemostatic pack** and apply **non-adherent dressing** and pads
- Prescribe **analgesia** and **laxatives**

37 Colostomy and Other Stomas

Matt Stephenson and Clare Byrne

Video | 5 min 16 s
Clare Byrne, Consultant General and Colorectal Surgeon
Lewisham Hospital, Lewisham
Filmed at the Royal Sussex County Hospital

Introduction

The laparotomy has been completed, the perforated rectosigmoid cancer or sigmoid diverticulitis has been identified, mobilised and heroically resected. The operation is finished. Well you would be forgiven for thinking so since your boss has taken off his gloves and walked off. If you're lucky, he'll have muttered to you instructions to make a colostomy and close up. **Happy you know how to proceed**?

That's just one kind of stoma—you've resected bowel but you're not happy to join the two ends together because there's a high chance they would leak, so you leave the distal end inside closed off and bring the other end out as an end stoma. If that end happens to be colon, like in a Hartmann's procedure, it's an **end colostomy**, if it's ileum, like in a subtotal colectomy, it's an **end ileostomy**.

There is of course another kind of stoma—a **loop colostomy** or **loop ileostomy**. Instead of bringing the end of a tube of gut out onto the surface of the abdominal wall, you bring out a tube of continuous bowel up to the surface of the abdominal wall and make a hole in it. If you put your finger in that hole, it could poke upstream or downstream.

You might make a **loop ileostomy** if you had just resected some rectum and made an anastomosis deep in the pelvis, but you weren't completely confident the anastomosis wasn't going to leak, you can't even inspect it properly it's so out of the way. Making an upstream (from the anastomosis) ileostomy diverts all the gastro-intestinal contents into a bag, and in the event of a leak may mitigate against its effects.

How to Operate: for MRCS Candidates and Surgical Trainees, First Edition. M. Stephenson. © 2011 John Wiley & Sons, Ltd. Published 2011 by John Wiley & Sons, Ltd.

A **loop colostomy**, however, would be made for a different reason. Imagine your 90-year-old patient has presented with a large bowel obstruction and your finger, or perhaps a CT, tells you they have an advanced obstructing rectal cancer and they're clearly not fit for a resection. Bowel obstruction and its ultimate consequence, a proximal perforation, or profuse vomiting and aspiration pneumonia is a horrible way to die. We can be much kinder. By simply lifting some proximal colon up to the abdominal wall and opening it out so the effluent ends up in a bag these nasty ends are prevented. It can even be done, as you'll see, through a hole the size of the stoma without any midline laparotomy scar.

In the **elective scenario** make sure the patient has been able to fully discuss the stoma and the implications of it with the **stoma care nurse**. The ideal site should also be **marked preoperatively**. In the **emergency situation** such luxuries are often not practical.

You may be making the colostomy at the end of having just done a laparotomy, or you may just be making a colostomy through a small trephine hole. There are two parts of the colon that are usually mobile enough to come up to the abdominal wall without tension—the **transverse colon** and the **sigmoid colon**. Therefore either choose a left lower quadrant site or right upper quadrant site (the hepatic flexure is lower than the splenic flexure so getting it on the right is easier).

In the event of having to decide for yourself which part of the bowel to bring out as a stoma, then the sigmoid, if mobile, does make a much better stoma than the transverse colon, which is generally not well tethered and does tend to prolapse and is difficult to manage.

This video shows a loop sigmoid colostomy, but the principles of stoma creation are similar and we will elaborate on any differences between this and the others.

Procedure

We'll begin by assuming you are solely making a stoma and that this isn't a stoma at the end of the operation—there's little difference but we'll come back to that in the Notes section.

Ideally, the patient is **supine** under **general anaesthetic** with the abdomen **shaved**, **prepped** and **draped**. NB It is possible to make a trephine colostomy under local anaesthesia if the patient is not fit for a general anaesthetic. If no mark has been made preoperatively you need to **identify a good location** for the stoma.

Firstly, it has to go through the rectus sheath, so it can't be too lateral. Secondly, it can't be too medial either or it will be in the way of any possible future midline laparotomy wound. Thirdly, it can't be too low where the patient can't easily reach it and see it but ideally low enough that high riding underwear will cover it. In patients with more protruberant abdomens it may need to be higher than in slim patients.

For a sigmoid colostomy (as in the video), if you imagine that McBurney's point is two-thirds of the way from umbilicus to ASIS, a reasonable rule of thumb is that the stoma should be about one-third of the way (and on the left obviously instead of the right). A transverse colostomy should be about halfway between the umbilicus and the right costal margin (it mustn't be too close to the costal margin).

Many people have their own pet ways of making a simple **circular hole** in the skin, roughly 4–5 cm in diameter. Some people make a freehand circle, some pick up the skin with forceps and cut round it. Another way is to make a cruciate incision, then pick up each corner of the four cut edges and incise the bases, making four quarters of a circle that you can then just cut off. You then need to **dissect** down through **superficial fascia** and **fat** down to the anterior rectus sheath. In general, there's no need to actually excise this fat unless there's a lot of it. Eventually, you'll come down onto **anterior rectus sheath**, which is a white fibrous layer. Make a **cruciate** incision in it. Beneath you'll see the vertically running **rectus abdominus**. **Retract** each side of this out of the way with Langenbeck retractors. Behind this muscle you will find the **posterior rectus sheath** and **peritoneum**. Pick these up in clips, check no bowel is caught in them and **open** the posterior rectus sheath and peritoneum together with scissors. Use your **fingers to stretch** this final layer—ideally for a

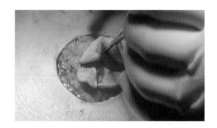

The circular hole has been made by an initial cruciate incision.

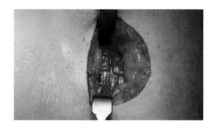

A cruciate incision has been made in the anterior rectus sheath, below it you see the rectus abdominus.

colostomy you would want to be able to admit four fingers, two for an ileostomy.

Fish around in the peritoneal cavity for large bowel—try to identify it by its **taenia coli** and **appendices epiploicae**. It should be right under your trephine. You may need to use Babcock forceps to encourage it out but take great care not to tear anything.

Once you've delivered a loop of colon out of the wound keep hold of an appendix epiploicae with the Babcock forceps just so it doesn't ping back into the abdomen whilst you're opening it (it shouldn't ping back by the way, that would suggest it's under tension which you don't want in a stoma, make sure

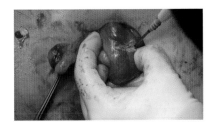

A transverse colostomy with diathermy (the edge tends to bleed a lot).

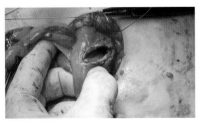

Note the large serosal bite taken by the stitch, an early prolapsing stoma with faeces going into the abdominal wall is a disaster.

there isn't something tethering it down or that you haven't picked up a very mobile caecum or transverse colon by mistake).

Make a **transverse incision** over the bowel with diathermy of about one-third of the circumference of the bowel. If the bowel looks like it's ready to explode with unpleasant faecal matter have a **sucker** ready. Take care not to suck too vigorously on the mucosa.

Suture the **edge of the hole** in the colon to the **skin of the wound** with **interrupted absorbable sutures** such as 2–0 Vicryl. This stitch needs to take **all layers** of the colon but, most importantly, a good bite of the strong **serosal** (outer) surface of the colon. The mucosa is the least important layer to include. It is also important to take a good (3 mm+) bite of the skin; separation of the stoma from the skin edge is not nice. Start by putting one stitch each at the north, south, east and west positions and then two or three in between each of these, a bit like the hours of a clock.

The colostomy is now made. Check you can easily **poke your finger in both limbs** of the loop without any obstruction

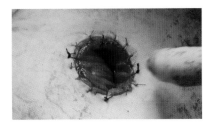

The finished product (sans stoma bag).

or kinking. **Clean** and **dry** the surrounding skin and **cut a hole** in the adhesive surface of the stoma bag to the size of the stoma. **Apply** the stoma bag.

Notes

In the event that you're making the stoma at the **end of a laparotomy**—this is easier in some ways as it's much more straightforward to find the bit of bowel to bring up to the surface. If you've just resected some bowel then the end will almost certainly have just been stapled off. Alternatively, you may be bringing out a loop of bowel to just divert the effluent. Either way, make sure that it can easily come up to the surface of the abdominal wall **without any tension and without being twisted**.

Proceed with **making the trephine** in just the same way as described above although you have the added advantage of knowing how far the bowel will reach and this can help you decide where to place the trephine. The fascial edges of the midline wound tend to retract laterally, it's sensible when making the trephine to pull on the fascial edge with Lanes forceps or similar so that it is at the same level as the skin or slightly further. This will mean that the skin hole for the stoma is at the same place as the fascial hole (a slight discrepancy is OK but a larger one will result in a kink in the stoma). The only difference between the end stoma and the loop stoma is that with the end stoma, you bring it out through the trephine and **cut off the staple line**—you make the stoma otherwise in exactly the same way.

There is only one **very important difference** between making a colostomy and an ileostomy. A colostomy is **flush** with the skin and an ileostomy needs to be **spouted**. Again there are many different methods for spouting an ileostomy.

One method is to take a serosal bite of the ileum, approximately 4 cm from the cut edge, then with the same needle take your bite at the cut edge of the bowel and then finally the skin bite. This needs to be done at the 4, 6 and 8 o clock positions, each time keep the suture material clipped without tying it. When all three stitches have been set up, tie them all, this should cause the edge of the stoma to evert. The remainder of the stitches can then be placed in the usual way, taking just skin and a single bite of bowel. When making a **loop ileostomy**, rather than an end, you only need to spout the afferent side, not the efferent side.

Summary

- The patient is under **general anaesthetic** with the abdomen **prepped** and **draped**
- Identify a **suitable site**
- Make a **circular skin incision**
- **Excise** the **skin**
- Dissect down to **anterior rectus sheath**
- **Open** anterior rectus sheath
- **Retract rectus abdominus**
- **Open posterior rectus sheath** and **peritoneum**
- **Deliver bowel**
- **Open bowel** and confirm **orientation**
- **Stitch bowel** to skin
- Apply **colostomy bag**

38 Small Bowel Resection and Anastomosis

Matt Stephenson and Jeremy S Clark

> **Video** | **16 min 19 s**
> Jeremy S Clark, Consultant Colorectal Surgeon
> Royal Sussex County Hospital, Brighton

Introduction

Small bowel always seems to be getting itself into **trouble**. Because it's suspended from a mesentery, its loops are **highly mobile**. This combined with its curiosity for tight enclosed spaces like **hernial sacs**, is a recipe for disaster.

Unlike its brother, the colon, loops of small bowel love sticking to other loops of small bowel, especially postoperatively, or to any intra-abdominal inflammatory patches, resulting in **adhesions** which can make the small bowel kink and obstruct the lumen. At other times it seems to commit hara-kiri for no apparent reason by twisting itself on its mesentery, a small bowel **volvulus**, resulting in first venous obstruction and consequent ischaemia. Its blood supply is also at threat from any **emboli** travelling down the aorta that decide to route off down the superior mesenteric artery.

Segments of it can become **inflamed**, usually as a result of Crohn's disease. Uncommonly, a primary **tumour** can arise from it, such as a small bowel lymphoma. More commonly however, other intra-abdominal malignancies spread transcoelomically, sending deposits onto the mesentery of the small bowel which can obstruct it.

It's not surprising therefore that you quite commonly have to rescue it, or, if the problem's gone too far, **resect** a segment and **join** the two ends together. In the scenario of small bowel incarcerated in a hernia, once it's reduced, assess it for **viability** after wrapping it in a swab soaked in warm saline. If it **pinks** up nicely, the serosa looks **shiny**, it's **peristalsing** and you can feel a **pulse** in the mesentery, don't resect it.

How to Operate: for MRCS Candidates and Surgical Trainees, First Edition. M. Stephenson. © 2011 John Wiley & Sons, Ltd. Published 2011 by John Wiley & Sons, Ltd.

If it's black or perforated it needs to come out. Anywhere in between requires experience and judgment, but usually it's pretty obvious. If in doubt, as a general rule, cut it out.

There are many ways of rejoining the ends back together again. The two principle categories being **stapled** or **hand sewn**. We've chosen to show the stapled method here, mainly because it's **quick**, very **safe** and **easy** to do, especially in the middle of the night. Whatever method you use, you must be mindful always of how disastrous an **anastomotic leak** (or **dehiscence**) can be, **meticulous attention** to the detail of each step is therefore essential. Fortunately, leaks from small bowel anastomoses happen uncommonly. The commonest reason for a leaking anastomosis is **ischaemia**. This tends to present itself most commonly **5–7 days postoperatively**. It can be because the resection margin you chose was too close to the ischaemic segment itself, or because it has become too ischaemic by the way the anastomosis has been fashioned; this guide will help you reduce the risk of that particular catastrophe.

Procedure

Lay the affected loop of small bowel out of the wound (a plus side to the mobility of the small bowel is that it's easy to deliver small bowel out of the wound) and clearly identify the **afferent** loop, the **efferent** loop and the **bit in between** that you want to cut out. You firstly want to identify **where to divide** the small bowel proximally and distally, your **resection**

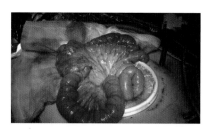

A loop of small bowel with a dilated afferent loop at the lower part of the picture leading onto the diseased segment and then distally, relatively collapsed small bowel. Ignore the white plastic ring—this is because this was part of a laparoscopic procedure.

margins, which should be far enough away from any ischaemic segment to look positively pink. **Inspect** the mesentery and look for the **mesenteric vessels;** you want to cut across the mesentery between the two resection points but by dividing as few of the major mesenteric vessels as possible.

Next, **open up the peritoneum** in a curved line between the two resection points by scoring along it with diathermy or scissors. You're roughly making a skewed semicircle. Don't make the apex of the semicircle too deep, that is away from the edge of the bowel as this will encroach on too many major mesenteric vessels which could be supplying the small bowel you want to anastomose. For benign disease you can keep the curve quite close to the bowel edge. Only cut the peritoneum—the most superficial layer of the mesentery—immediately below this are the mesenteric vessels often surrounded by a lot of fat.

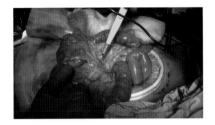

The diathermy finger switch is scoring along the peritoneum over the mesentery.

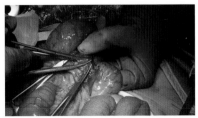

Mesenteric vessels are clipped.

Once the peritoneum is divided you can much more clearly see the mesenteric vessels. Using scissors **create a window** between the vessels by opening and closing the blades, and then **another window** a short distance from the other window. **Clip and divide** the vessels in between your windows. **Ligate** the vessels firmly using an absorbable suture such as Vicryl 2–0, or 0 for the bigger vessels (you can save time by only putting two throws on the side that you're resecting). Keep making further windows all the way along your mesenteric curve, and ligate and divide all the vessels in between.

You will then find you have one big mesenteric window beside the segment

of small bowel to be resected. You'll see that a **transition point** develops in the small bowel between the normal bowel and the bowel that you've just devascularised, which is becoming very dusky indeed. You'll then be able to clearly see where you would like your anastomotic edges to be—**choose a level** of small bowel a short distance from the dusky edge. **Lay** the afferent and efferent loops **next to each other**. You are going to make a **side-to-side anastomosis**. Although it is physically one side of bowel next to one side of bowel, **functionally** it is an **end-to-end anastomosis**. The

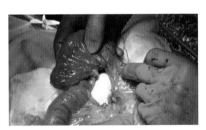

The mesentery is fully divided over the affected segment of small bowel. A clear transition point between viable and ischaemic small bowel is visible at the distal end.

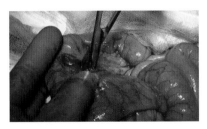

A window is made in the mesentery in an avascular area.

loops must come together **without any tension**. If there are adhesions restricting the mobility of the bowel, these must be divided.

You are about to open small bowel; **protect the wound** by laying some large swabs underneath your anastomosis site in case of spillage. Some people also use non-crushing **small bowel clamps**, especially if the afferent end is very distended and likely to spill everywhere upon opening (in which case also have a sucker ready). Using diathermy, make a small **enterotomy** about 0.5–1.0 cm away from your chosen resection level on both afferent and efferent ends of bowel, on the **antimesenteric** border. **Insert** one half of **the stapler** through one enterotomy and the other half down the other enterotomy. Bring these halves together so they **engage** with each other. Check the bowel **isn't twisted** and that nothing else has got **trapped** in the jaws of the stapler. **Fully close** the stapler and once you're happy with one final check that the bowel's not twisted and no extraneous material is caught up, **slide the stapling mechanism** all the way—this will fire **four parallel rows of staples**, with rows 1 and 3 offset against rows 2 and 4. Then **retract the sliding mechanism**—this will run a **blade** between the staples leaving two rows on each side. The two loops are therefore joined together. Of course you haven't yet severed the undesirable segment of small bowel. Next pick up the **edges of the enterotomies** with one pair of **Babcock forceps** and

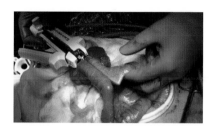

The two arms of the stapler have been passed down the limbs of the small bowel to form the lumen of the anastomosis.

hold these up. **Refill** the stapling device and **staple** across the two loops of small bowel just proximal to the enterotomies, that is **perpendicular** to the direction of the previous stapling. Send the specimen for **histopathological assessment**.

The small bowel is usually perfused by an anastomosis of blood vessels. Ordinarily, if you choose any one single point on the small bowel, blood can come towards it from any angle. However, now you've divided it, right at the divided edge blood can only come from one direction, and even that blood has to negotiate its way through the staple line. This means that there is a small risk of the very edge becoming ischaemic. Most people therefore **oversew** the distal staple line to create a back up layer in case it does. You can use a **continuous running suture** catching just the **seromuscular** layer on each side **inverting both corners**. A non-braided suture such as polydioxanone (**PDS**) runs smoothly through the tissue and is ideal for this. You are not including the staple line in your suture, this will only make the edge even more

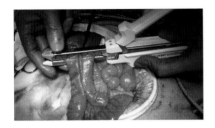

The final staple line to close off the anastomosis and remove the specimen.

ischaemic, you are inverting the staple line. Now if the edge does become ischaemic and break down, there is another back up layer of strength.

Where the two limbs of the small bowel have been stapled together, there is an **angle** which looks as though it could easily come apart. Most people therefore make an **additional single interrupted suture** between both limbs for support.

The final issue is whether to **close the mesenteric window** you initially created. The rationale for doing this is so a loop of small bowel **can't herniate** through it. The rationale for not doing this is that by stitching each edge of the mesenteric window, you **risk catching the mesenteric vessels** which can cause ischaemia to your anastomosis. If the window is only tiny it's reasonable to leave it. If it's very large, it's also reasonable to leave it—it's less likely bowel will get trapped through a big defect (in the same way as very large incisional hernias rarely become irreducible) and more likely you'll cause ischaemia by all the sutures required to close it. If it's somewhere in between then close it but only stitch together the edges of the defect where you have already tied off vessels, or just stitch the thin peritoneal layers together. Put the bowel back into the abdomen.

Summary

- **Lay out** the small bowel
- Identify the **afferent** and **efferent** loops with the diseased segment in between
- Identify the **resection margins**
- **Open the peritoneum** in a curved line
- **Ligate** and **divide** the **mesenteric vessels**
- Re-identify the **healthy resection margins**
- **Lay** the two loops **next to each other** and check for tension
- **Protect the wound** from spillage +/− bowel clamps
- Make **enterotomies**
- **Insert** jaws of **stapler**
- **Fire stapling mechanism**
- **Pick up** edges of **enterotomies** with Babcock forceps
- **Fire second line** of staples perpendicular to last
- Send specimen to **histopathology**
- **Oversew** staple line
- Insert additional **supporting suture**
- **Return bowel** to abdomen

39 Excision of Pilonidal Sinus

Matt Stephenson and Stephen Whitehead

> **Video** | **4 min 22 s**
> Stephen Whitehead, Consultant General Surgeon
> Conquest Hospital, St Leonards-on-Sea

Introduction

You'll encounter pilonidal disease either as an emergency in the case of an **acute abscess** or electively for a **troublesome sinus** that may keep flaring up into an abscess, or it may be chronically discharging.

In the case of an acute abscess, **incise and drain it** in just the same way as you would for any other abscess (see *Incision and Drainage of Abscess* Chapter 4) but warn the patient that they may not have heard the last from their pilonidal disease. You haven't after all removed the source of the problem; half of them will go on to need further surgery for their pilonidal disease. For a sinus the management is different, you want to excise the sinus completely, not just drain it.

There is much discussion about the different options for what to do once you've completely excised it—do you close it? How would you close it? Leave it open? Marsupialise it? Create a flap to cover the defect? Well it all gets very complicated and frankly quite boring, unless that's your thing. Generally speaking, in the presence of sepsis or extensive sinuses making skin closure impossible without excessive tension, it's best to leave the wound open to heal by second intention. If there is no or minimal sepsis and only a small sinus, then get those wounds together to close primarily.

Procedure

With the patient under **general anaesthetic**, turn the patient **prone**. It's much easier to operate on a horizontal surface than a vertical one (you don't drop quite so many swabs on the floor). If there is a substantial amount of fat on the buttocks and you seem to be peering down into a

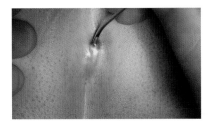

The probe has been inserted into the larger sinus opening.

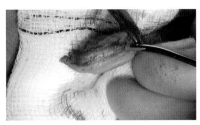

The specimen is being probed to check the whole sinus has been excised.

deep cavern, **tape** each buttock to the table on each side. **Shave**, **prep** and **drape** in the usual way.

Whilst you can see some midline pits you can't be entirely clear from inspection alone what lies beneath. The most useful way of exploring what's what is with a **probe**. Insert that into any of the pits and see where it goes. Usually the pits all communicate with each other in the midline, but you may find **lateral extensions** of the sinus.

Excise the **whole sinus** as an **ellipse** taking a very narrow rim of normal tissue all around it. Pilonidal sinuses tend to **bleed** quite a lot so diathermy is essential. Some sinuses point right down deep towards **sacral fascia** whereas some lie just under the skin. The probing will help determine this. Either way, it's better to go a little deeper to fully excise the sinus than leave it there to recur in the future. **Inspect** the wound bed and look for evidence of side branches of sinuses. These appear as little **granulation rosettes** and if you probe them you may identify a further track, in which case excise all around this too.

Once you're happy you've eliminated the sinus tracks, decide whether you're going to **close the wound primarily** or **leave it open**. If there's been no pus and the cavity is quite small thus the wound edges come together without tension, it's reasonable to close it primarily. You can use deep absorbable sutures to get the deep layers together and then separate interrupted skin sutures, or you could use **mattress sutures**. If you're faced with a large cavity or if there was active infection, **leave it all open** and dress it, as is. It will have to heal by **second intention**. The cavity will fill up with **granulation tissue** which will then be **epithelialised** over. This can take **2 to 3 months** and is very labour intensive on the part of the nursing

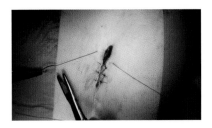

Primary closure with vertical mattress sutures.

staff. One of the advantages to the primary closure is that if the wound appears to be getting infected, it's easy to just take out the sutures, reverting essentially to plan B, and leaving the wound open.

Notes

Bear in mind that most pilonidal abscesses do not develop in the midline where the pits are. In the midline the skin is too tethered to the sacral fascia to accommodate such a thing, instead most pilonidal abscesses are just off the midline.

There is another category of options if trying to close the defect: **skin flaps**. These can work very well when used for the right cases, but can be disastrous if you don't get it right and the flaps necrose leaving you with a much bigger defect than you had originally. They involve swinging a flap of skin from the adjacent area to the midline, there are various types. They are generally reserved for recurrent pilonidal disease. One final option is to marsupialise it which means to stitch the skin edge down to the sacral fascia. This has the effect of making a deep cavity much shallower, thus reducing the size of the wound that needs to heal by second intention.

One final note, is that when you do close by primary closure, there is evidence to say that closing the wound in the midline heals slower than if you close it just off the midline. To do that, you actually have to take your skin ellipse slightly off centre. In this video, the sinus was so small, we could get away with a midline closure.

Summary

- The patient is **prone** under **general anaesthetic**
- **Shave**, **prep** and **drape**
- **Explore** the sinus(es) with a **probe**
- **Excise** all diseased tissue as a **skin ellipse**
- Check for **further branches** of the sinus
- Either **close up** or **leave open**

40 Right Hemicolectomy

Matt Stephenson and Peter J Webb

> **Video** | **26 min 44 s**
> Peter J Webb, Consultant General and Colorectal Surgeon
> Medway Maritime Hospital, Gillingham

Introduction

Sooner or later during your early surgical years, you will be judged on whether or not you can do a right hemicolectomy. It's probably the first kind of bowel surgery you'll do, and also the first major abdominal case. It is therefore a **milestone operation** and your ability to do one or not is often used, albeit arbitrarily, as a marker of how you're getting on in your training.

Miserably, at the moment, you may well find yourself working for a boss who is just learning to do them **laparoscopically**. Unfortunately, you are unlikely to get to do much so if open right hemicolectomies are a rarity in your hospital, consider it your number one priority to get your hands on any that come up.

The commonest indication, of course, for a right hemicolectomy is **carcinoma** of the ascending colon or in the case of an **extended right hemicolectomy**, of the transverse colon. That means getting a good clearance of **lymph nodes** and at least **5 cm** each side of the tumour is imperative. In benign cases such as **caecal volvulus** (a great learning case because the colon's very mobile, already making it an easy operation) or **terminal ileitis** these margins aren't an issue.

Procedure

With the patient **supine** under **general anaesthetic** the abdomen is **shaved**, **prepped** and **draped**. There are **two options** for the skin incision. You could just do a simple **midline laparotomy** centred equally above and below the umbilicus. Or, you could make a **transverse incision**. Both incisions are about the same length but the advantages of the transverse incision is that it tends to be **less painful** postoperatively—**fewer dermatomes** are cut through and the incision doesn't move as much with respiration as with the upper part of a midline (and also escape the

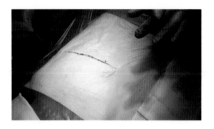

A transverse incision has been made just above the umbilicus.

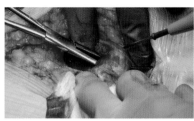

Artery forceps are elevating part of the rectus abdominus to be divided.

epidural). A transverse scar is also **cosmetically** far better on the abdomen. You have to be **sure** however that it is a right hemicolectomy you are doing, that is you have **confirmed malignancy** seen on **colonoscopy** and **three-dimensional imaging** (such as CT)—don't trust the colonoscopy to tell you where it is. If you open up and find it's not going to be a right hemicolectomy you may well struggle through your wound. It can be extended to the other side if absolutely necessary but you are then cutting through a lot of muscle. Don't use a transverse incision in an emergency for these reasons.

Assuming you've opted for the transverse incision (see the *Laparotomy* Chapter 9 for the midline), make a **transverse** incision going laterally from just above or below the **umbilicus** to about the **anterior axillary line**. Cut through **superficial fascia** and **fat**, down onto the **external oblique** laterally and **rectus sheath** medially. **Cut** right through both of these using diathermy, elevating the rectus abdominus with large

artery forceps or similar—the **inferior epigastric artery** may need to be ligated. Again using **diathermy** cut through the internal oblique and transversus. When you're doing this you do tend to feel that you're being terribly destructive to the tissues, not like the relatively non-destructive muscle splitting of the Lanz approach for an appendicectomy, for example, but they heal well anyway and are less painful—just stitch them back up well at the end. Behind the rectus abdominus you'll find the **posterior rectus sheath** with **peritoneum** closely adherent behind it.

So get **two clips** on the posterior rectus sheath and peritoneum together, feel between them with finger and thumb to ensure there's nothing adherent to the inner surface, and **open it** with scissors. You'll then see that beautiful little black hole appear in the peritoneum—you've entered the peritoneal cavity. Slide your **finger in** and check nothing's adherent to the inner surface and then open up the peritoneum in the line of the incision.

Examine the abdomen in just the same way as you would for a midline approach. Aside from examining the liver for spread, one of the most important things you want to do is **examine the colon** to find exactly where the tumour is and to be sure there are no other **synchronous tumours** elsewhere. Imagine doing a right hemicolectomy and making an anastomosis which then blows because of another obstructing distal lesion. It's happened. Also once you've found the tumour, don't **over handle** it, you only risk seeding malignant cells elsewhere. Many people advocate leaving examination of the tumour itself until last for this reason.

Your transverse wound is at a level roughly half way up the ascending colon, which means it's usually pretty easy to access all of it by a combination of good retraction and manipulation of the right colon. A self-retaining retractor, such as **Golligher retractors**, is often helpful. From here on in, the operation is just the same as for the midline approach.

Assuming your intraoperative findings are consistent with your preoperative assessment—get on with the operation. The **first manoeuvre** is to have your assistant **retract the right lateral** abdominal wall, with a **Morris retractor** say, whilst you **hold the caecum** in your non-dominant hand **pulling it medially**. This opens up the **right paracolic gutter**, and in there is the key to the operation. You are looking for the **magical white line of Toldt**. Where the

peritoneum covering the ascending colon folds around to meet the peritoneum of the lateral abdominal wall, there you will see a **white line**. It runs all the way up from the **caecum** to the **hepatic flexure**, it's more obvious in some people than others, and becomes particularly difficult to see if the tissues are infiltrated with fat. With your assistant maintaining lateral retraction and you pulling the caecum towards you (holding it with a swab helps to stop it slipping) the white line is **under tension**. **Cut it**. You can use scissors or diathermy. As it opens up you will find **loose areolar tissue** between the colon and the posterior abdominal wall. This plane is God's gift to surgeons. Once you're in it, the colon quite rapidly comes up into your hand and it's a surprisingly **bloodless** plane too. Continue along the white line cutting all the way up to the hepatic flexure and continue the **dissection** through the loose areolar tissue by a combination of sharp and blunt dissection, until the whole of the ascending colon is **mobilised** up out of the wound

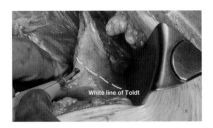

The lateral peritoneal reflection of the ascending colon is being divided along the white line of Toldt, which can be difficult to see if there's lots of fat.

into your hand. If, as in the case in the video, the tumour is adherent to the parietal peritoneum of the pelvic or abdominal side wall, cut just around this outside of the usual plane thus removing the tumour *en bloc*.

Regarding the top and the bottom of the ascending colon, you need to continue the mobilisation a little way into the mesentery of the **terminal ileum** and this is done in just the same way but the white line is not so obvious; you can continue in the same direction though, mobilising a little of the terminal ileum. At the **hepatic flexure**, you will also need to divide any other tissue that seems to be suspending the colon. So pull this time with **downwards traction** on the hepatic flexure and divide any of this tissue in the same way under the liver. You then need to continue the mobilisation of the proximal transverse colon. This is best done by sliding your finger around behind the tissue suspending the transverse colon close to the hepatic flexure—which will consist of gastrocolic omentum and transverse mesocolon—and cutting down onto this.

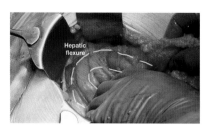

Now viewing from below, up into the right upper quadrant, the hepatic flexure can be seen.

An alternative approach is to work your way up the ascending colon as described above and then start dissecting from the transverse colon back towards the hepatic flexure, eventually joining up at the hepatic flexure. This is particularly useful if it's a difficult, deep hepatic flexure. First, choose how far along the transverse colon you want to get your anastomosis. Let's say it's one-third of the way along. Next, **dissect a hole** in the **gastrocolic omentum** (not too close to the stomach—don't forget the **gastroepiploic arteries** run there) and see if a cavity quickly opens up. If it does, you've probably just entered the **lesser sac**. You can then put your finger in it and hold up the gastrocolic omentum all the way back to the hepatic flexure and **divide it** by applying **haemostatic clips** and dividing in between. If, however, no such space exists and you seem to keep digging, then you will probably end up going straight through the transverse mesocolon which has joined it from behind (to confirm which space you're in, flip the colon superiorly and look to see if you've gone straight through the other side of the transverse mesocolon). This is not a problem, you need to divide it anyway to resect the lateral bit of the transverse colon. So whatever the particular arrangement in your patient, divide these mesenteries so that the right colon is fully mobilised up to the proximal transverse colon.

As you are completing your mobilisation of the right colon, you need to be aware

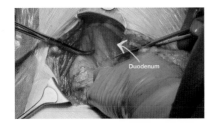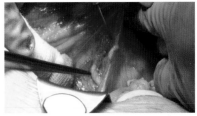

The right colon has been mobilised and retracted medially to reveal the duodenum and the right ureter (viewing from below).

of **three structures** to avoid: the **duodenum** is right under there and you don't want to injure this, you really don't, so take great care. There is also the **ureter**, which isn't always seen in a right hemicolectomy and you don't necessarily have to go hunting for it as you should in a left hemicolectomy, but be mindful of it. The same for the third thing to be on the look out for—the **gonadal vessels** which bleed if you prang them.

Next you need to deal with the **blood supply**. You're holding up the mobilised ascending colon with your hand but it's still attached to the posterior abdominal wall by a mesentery (a mesentery you've created by mobilising it because it was originally plastered to the posterior abdominal wall, i.e. it **was** retroperitoneal) which contains the **right colic** and **ileocolic arteries**. Identify your point on the small bowel where you've mobilised up to and **score across** the **peritoneal surface** with scissors or diathermy, taking just the peritoneum, up to your chosen point on the transverse colon. Remember that if this is for cancer, you want to take

as many of the local lymph nodes as possible, therefore arc the division of the mesentery proximally towards the root of the vessels. Through careful dissection **identify the major vessels**, and **ligate**

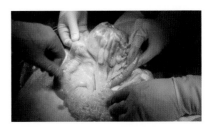

The mobilised right colon is held up on its mesentery, which is displayed nicely to identify the major vessels for ligation.

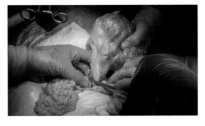

The ileocolic has been clipped with large artery forceps for transfixion.

and **divide** them. In this way, **divide all** of the mesentery so that the terminal portion of ileum, entire right colon and proximal transverse colon aren't attached to anything except being in continuity as a tube with the rest of the bowel. You should also include in your resection the **omentum** hanging down from the front of the proximal transverse colon, this usually mean splitting the omentum at the chosen level of transverse colon resection, leaving the left side of the omentum be.

Bring the ileum and the transverse colon together **side by side** and check they're not under any **tension**. Avoiding tension in the anastomosis is absolutely crucial, and may require further mobilisation of the ileum, they do however usually come together without much persuasion. By this stage the end of the ileum and the proximal transverse colon are going to start looking very **dusky** as you just divided their blood supply. This line of **demarcation** helps you know precisely where to make the anastomosis. You want to be well clear of any duskiness. So lay the healthy ileum and healthy transverse colon side by side. Apply a proximal **non-crushing bowel clamp** to the ileum and one to the transverse colon. Lay **large swabs** beneath the bowel to protect the wound from contamination.

You can make the anastomosis either **stapled** or **hand sewn**. In the video you'll see a hand sewn anastomosis—the stapled one is essentially identical to that seen in the *Small Bowel Resection and Anastomosis* video, Chapter 38 (so you don't feel you've missed out)**, but to describe it again: open** the ileum and the transverse colon on their **anti-mesenteric** borders with diathermy to make a **small hole** in the first part of healthy bowel. Take your **linear stapling device** and pass **one-half** of the stapler down the hole in the **ileum going proximally** and the other down the hole in the **colon going distally**. Bring the anti-mesenteric borders of the ileum and colon together so that the stapler components **engage** with each other. Make sure that you haven't got **anything else caught behind** and that you **aren't twisting** either the ileum or the colon. Once you're happy, advance the **sliding mechanism** which inserts **two rows of staples** all the way along and then **withdraw it**, thus cutting between the two rows of staples, making your **anastomosis**.

Now **grip the edge** of the hole the stapler just came out of, with **Babcock forceps**, front and back and **elevate them**. You can now get a **stapler refill** and staple across at **90 degrees** to the last stapler through both colon and ileum, just below the Babcock forceps thus amputating the specimen (to be put in a histopathology bucket with formaldehyde) along with the first stapler hole (sometimes if the two bits of bowel together are quite wide you'll need to do this in two separate goes with a second refill). **Feel** the anastomosis between finger and thumb for **patency**. Check all the bowel **looks healthy**, if it's starting to get dusky, you're going to have to resect a bit

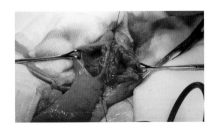

The outer, seromuscular layer of the back row has been inserted, this will be followed by an inner full thickness layer.

through it at some stage in the future, it's best to close it, but take great care to only take small bites of the peritoneum—don't take deep bites that could catch blood vessels going to your anastomosis.

Wash the abdomen out to remove any contamination or blood clots and check for **haemostasis**. **Close** the transverse incision with **mass closure** as you would for the midline, and say a prayer for your anastomosis.

further back to healthy bowel and do the anastomosis again. Which is really annoying at 3 am. Some people like to then **oversew** the staple line, at least inverting the stapled corners.

For the hand sewn anastomosis, this is essentially identical to the gastro-jejunostomy seen in the *Gastrectomy* Chapter 25, so check this for details or watch the video. One crucial difference with the stapled anastomosis is that rather than laying the two sides together and then stapling them, you just staple the bowel at each end of the specimen aligning the stapler roughly perpendicular to the bowel and then suture them together.

Either way you anastomose, you leave a large mesenteric window. Some people close this and others leave it. In general, if you could imagine bowel herniating

Notes

In the event that the indication for the surgery is obstruction in the emergency setting, there is debate about whether or not to perform an **anastomosis** or to bring the two ends out as a **double-barrelled stoma**. In this case you're making a very large oedematous, and possibly hypertrophied, small bowel anastomose onto collapsed colon. The rate of leaks in emergency right hemi-colectomies is considerably higher than with elective cases. Some units adopt a policy of a double-barrelled stoma for all emergency right hemicolectomies, which can then theoretically be reversed later. If in doubt about the quality of the bowel ends, bring them out as a stoma. Much better to have a live patient with a reversible stoma than a dead one with a leak from a heroic anastomosis.

Summary

- The patient is **supine** under **general anaesthetic**
- The abdomen is **shaved**, **prepped** and **draped**
- Make a **midline** or **right transverse** incision
- **Examine** the abdominal contents
- **Locate** the tumour
- Divide **Toldt's white line**
- **Mobilise** the right colon **medially**
- **Mobilise** the terminal **ileum** and hepatic flexure
- Divide the **mesentery** of the right colon **ligating** all the vessels
- Bring the healthy **colon and ileum together** and make a **small hole** in each
- **Insert the jaws** of the stapler and **staple** them together
- Staple a second time at **90 degrees** to the first **across ileum and colon**
- **Oversew** the staple line if desired
- Or perform a **hand sewn anastomosis**
- **Wash out** if contaminated, ensure haemostasis
- **Mass closure**

41 Surgical Instruments

Matt Stephenson and Cheryl Funnell

> **Video** | **37 min 17 s**
> Cheryl Funnell, Lead Practitioner, General and
> Emergency Team and Registered Nurse
> Conquest Hospital, St Leonards-on-Sea

Introduction

So many things in surgery are never actually taught; you will just be expected to pick them up by osmosis during your time in theatre. Learning the names of surgical instruments is one of those things. There is no secret course or lecture you've missed, it simply doesn't get taught to trainee surgeons. Yet it sounds so much more professional to ask for Gillies forceps rather than 'some tweezers'.

One of the big problems with learning the names of instruments is that some hospitals call certain instruments one thing whilst others call it something else; this is usually the case at least with scissors and forceps. There is little continuity between units, sometimes even day surgery will call an instrument one thing and the main theatres, another—all in the same hospital. However, you can turn this to your advantage; you can quite easily make up any name you like, who are they to say you're wrong? OK perhaps not.

Some have eponymous names, others simply are called what they are. Even if you don't learn the eponymous names (if there is one), learn how to describe the instrument, for example long dissecting scissors versus stitch-cutting scissors. We have used here some of the more commonly used names, but in your own hospital they may very well be different.

There is such a vast array of instruments they can't all be covered here. The best way to learn each of their names and what their special powers are, is to spend some time with an experienced scrub person.

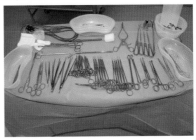

A minor basic general set.

How to Operate: for MRCS Candidates and Surgical Trainees, First Edition. M. Stephenson. © 2011 John Wiley & Sons, Ltd.
Published 2011 by John Wiley & Sons, Ltd.

Commonly used general instruments

Rampley sponge holder

The **Rampley sponge holder** is frequently used to hold a swab, which can be used to prep the skin and then be discarded. You can also wrap a swab around its jaws and use this to dissect or dab blood—the so called **'swab-on-a-stick'**. It's also useful in its own right to grasp hold of the gallbladder and pull it this way and that.

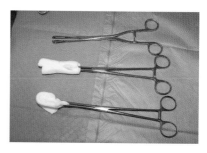

Above down, the 'nude' Rampleys; swab-on-a-stick; swab mounted for prepping.

Forceps

Forceps vary, firstly, on whether they are **toothed** or **non-toothed**. Toothed forceps are good to grasp the skin edge when closing the subcuticular layer but never use them in the abdomen where you risk making an enterotomy—non-toothed forceps are much safer for this. Secondly, they vary in their length and robustness. The average toothed forceps common to many sets are **Gillies forceps** (although you can get non-toothed versions) whereas **McIndoe**

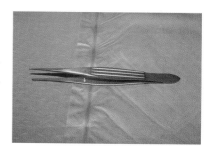

McIndoe (non-toothed) forceps.

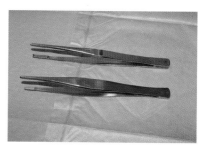

Lanes forceps.

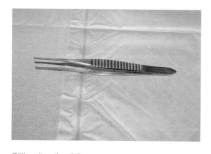

Gillies (toothed) forceps.

forceps (sometimes called **DeBakey forceps**) are common non-toothed options. **Lanes forceps** can be toothed or non-toothed and are a little larger.

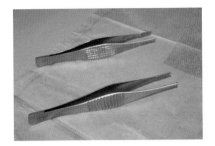

Ramsey forceps.

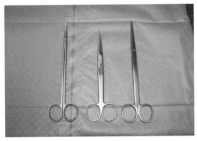

Left, McIndoe scissors; middle and right, different lengths of Mayo scissors.

More robust tips, for grabbing hold of firmer material such as tendons or cartilage are **Ramsey forceps**.

Scissors

Scissors broadly speaking are divided into **dissecting scissors** (such as **McIndoe scissors**) and **stitch-cutting scissors** (such as **Mayo scissors**). You shouldn't use the former to cut stitches because it blunts the blades, and you shouldn't use the latter to dissect as they aren't delicate enough. Sometimes there is tough tissue to cut through, however, such as when opening the abdomen, and here using the

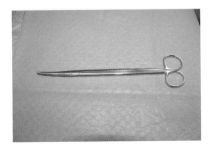

McIndoe dissecting scissors.

Mayo scissors to chomp through the linea alba, once the bowel is out of the way, is the preferred method for some. They can also be used on tough scar tissue. Dissecting scissors are almost always curved as this makes dissecting easier. Mayo scissors can be curved or straight.

Haemostatic clips

You'll need something to clamp off vessels, or bits of tissue in which you think there is a vessel. You need a haemostatic clip, or clamp, or more confusingly also generally called artery forceps. They range in size, can be straight or curved, and can be slender or thicker. **Mosquito** or **Dunhill artery forceps** are on the smaller side. **Spencer–Wells artery forceps** are average in length but quite slender whereas **Birkett artery forceps** are fatter and more robust for grasping chunks of tissue. Going up in size are **Roberts artery forceps** and even bigger for fat chunks of tissue deep in the abdomen for instance, **Moynihan artery forceps**.

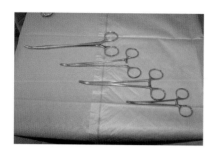

From above down, Roberts, Spencer Wells, Birkett and Dunhill–Artery forceps.

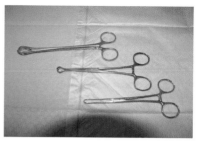

Above down, Lanes tissue-holding forceps, Babcock forceps and Allis forceps.

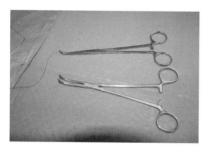

Lahey artery forceps.

Lahey artery forceps have a right angle turn on their tips. This makes them very useful to dissect around the back of vessels or ducts, and you can also mount a tie on them and pass it easily around an inaccessible vessel in order to ligate it.

Special tissue-holding forceps

There are three particularly special tissue-holding forceps (the names of which you'll be glad to know are usually quite consistent across the land and therefore worth memorising). **Babcock forceps** have atraumatic tips that are excellent

for encircling the appendix or picking up bowel or other tissue. Atraumatic should really be in apostrophes—they **can** damage the serosal surface of the bowel, so when fishing around for the caecum in an appendicectomy—still be careful. **Allis forceps** are perfect for picking up the subcuticular layer of skin to retract or lift it up, or to place on some tissue that you're resecting and want to draw it up into the wound. Beware however, these cannot be used on bowel—they will damage it. Then there's the **Lanes tissue holding forceps** (not to be

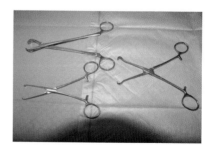

Top left, Lanes tissue-holding forceps; bottom left, Allis forceps; right, Babcock forceps.

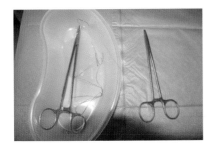

Needle holders.

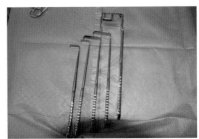

Increasing sizes of Langenbeck retractors from left to right, with a Morris retractor far right.

confused with Lanes forceps)—with very much traumatic tips, they will grasp anything firmly by biting into it, so these should only be used on structures such as the fascia of the abdominal wall—never inside the abdomen.

Needle holders

Needle holders, like everything else, vary depending on the length and the robustness of the tip. Clearly, a small needle requires a fine tip, a big needle requires a robust tip. A deep suture requires a long needle holder, a skin suture requires a shorter one. If the handles are golden, the tips are made from **tungsten carbide**—a very strong needle holder that won't slip.

Retractors

Retractors can be either of the kind that you pull on, or that holds itself apart, that is self-retaining. Probably the commonest example of the former are **Langenbeck retractors**—excellent for retracting the edge of a wound—and come in a variety of sizes. An alternative is the **Czerny retractors**, which has two prongs to lift

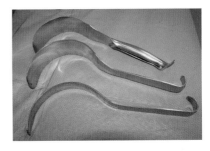

Varying shapes and sizes of Deaver retractors.

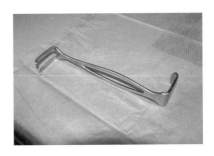

Czerny retractor.

up the skin edge. To retract the abdominal wall you need something more robust like a **Morris retractor** or to retract deeper layers, a **Deaver retractor**.

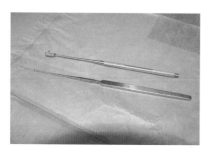

Above, McIndoe double-prong skin hook; below, Gillies skin hook.

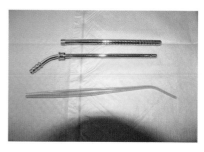

Above, Pooles sucker with guard; below, Yankauer sucker.

Sometimes you only need to retract the skin edge, when creating a flap for instance in a mastectomy or thyroidectomy. An instrument with a single hook is a **Gillies skin hook**, and with two hooks, a **McIndoe double-prong skin hook**.

The commonest and most 'middle-sized' **self-retaining retractor** is a **Travers retractor**. For a deeper wound, use a very similar instrument—the **Norfolk and Norwich retractor**. For a small version, for instance for a temporal artery biopsy, you can use a **West retractor**.

Left, Norfolk and Norwich retractor; right, Travers retractor.

Suckers

You're going to want to keep the operative site dry from all that blood you keep spilling . . . A **Yankauer sucker** is a plastic disposable sucker that sucks from the tip and is thus useful when you want to suck in a particularly focal place. Often you may just want to suck more blindly in a pool of fluid, or if the tip keeps getting blocked up with lumps of fat, in which case you can use a **Pooles sucker**, which has an inner piece and an outer guard which screws onto it. It sucks over a broad surface area. Using just the inner piece can be a useful instrument for doing blunt dissection.

Diathermy equipment

Sucking up the blood isn't going to stop it bleeding though unfortunately, for that you may find the diathermy helpful. Diathermy comes in two broad kinds:

Monopolar—the AC current passes from a diathermy machine, through a lead to a diathermy instrument usually either forceps, a finger switch or

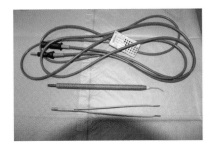

Above, diathermy lead; middle, diathermy point; below, diathermy forceps.

pointpasses through the tissue you want to coagulate or cut, through the patient's body, then through the earthing plate, then through a wire and back to the diathermy machine. Never use it on an extremity or the returning current to the earthing plate will concentrate at the narrowest point and heat upa lot.

Bipolar the AC current passes between two metal components of the instrument, for examples the tips of some forceps or the blades of some scissors. It passes from one tip, through the tissue to be cut or coagulated and back up to the machine through the other tip (thus also having the advantage of going nowhere near the patient's pacemaker).

It is strongly recommended that you always ensure that the smoke produced from burning flesh, also known as the diathermy plume, is extracted by an evacuation device, because of the potentially oncogenic contents.

Miscellaneous general

Pledgets are small, usually made of gauze, almost pea sized things which can be grasped in the end of a **Kocher forceps** (the only useful role for such forceps as they have an extremely traumatic bite to the tip of them). These can be very useful for fine blunt dissection, for instance when trying to define the structures in Calot's triangle or the axilla.

Bowel clamps can be **non-crushing (Doyen)** and **crushing (Stevens)**, curved or straight. Never use crushing bowel clamps unless you're planning on removing whatever bit of bowel you're crushing, and sending it off to the lab.

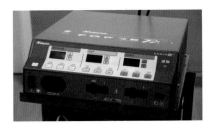

A diathermy machine.

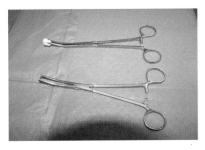

Kocher forceps with and without a pledget.

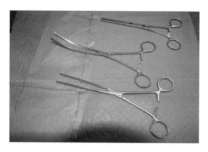

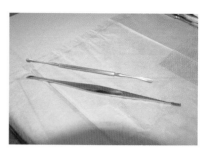

Above, crushing bowel clamp, middle and bottom, curved and straight non-crushing bowel clamps.

Top, Howarth elevator; bottom, McDonald dissector.

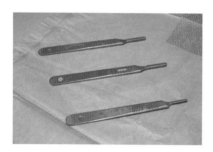

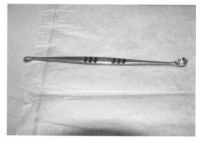

Bard–Parker handles.

Volkmann spoon.

Blades are mounted on **Bard-Parker handles**, or colloquially known as **BP handles**. They come in a variety of sizes.

The **Howarth elevator** and the **McDonald dissector** have a variety of uses. They can help in bluntly dissecting a plane, for instance during an endarterectomy or lifting up the nasal mucosa.

The **Volkmann spoon** is a type of curette; they come in various sizes and can be used to scrape out, for instance the lining of an abscess cavity or sinus, or larger ones to scrape out the femoral canal.

Orthopaedic

Bone spikes and **ring-handled spikes** are useful to get control of fragments of bone when operating on a fracture site for instance.

Northfield bone nibblers come in a variety of sizes and do the function you'd expect—nibble bits of bone—useful for anything from nibbling off osteophytes to removing residual bony spikes in a toe amputation. **Bailey bone cutters** are the bony version of scissors and also come in a variety of sizes.

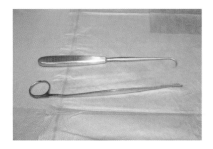

Above, bone spike; bottom, ring-handled spike.

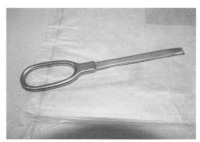

Bristow periosteal elevator.

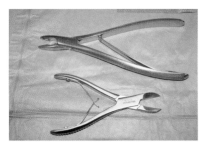

Above, Northfield bone nibbler; below, Bailey bone cutter.

An **orthopaedic mallet** can be used for chiseling, banging home prosthetic hips and generally making a lot of noise.

Remember bone is covered in a layer of periosteum, which you frequently need to peel off the bone cortex itself. The **Bristow periosteal elevator** will do this for you nicely.

ENT

The **dental syringe** has greater versatility than just invoking fear at a visit to the dentists. It stores a glass vial, the contents of which can be inserted into mucous membranes of the nose or mouth.

The **toffee hammer** is the much more genteel version of the orthopaedic mallet. It's light and easily handled and can be

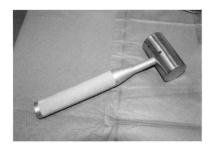

Orthopaedic mallet.

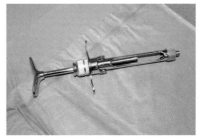

Dental syringe.

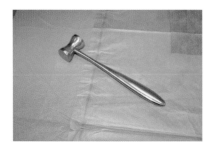

Toffee hammer.

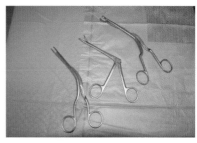

Left, nasal scissors; middle, Tilley–Henkel forceps; right, nasal polyp forceps.

used for instance to chisel up the nasal carriage.

Tilley-Henkel forceps can be used to extract tissue deep within the nasal cavity and beyond. There are a variety of other **nasal polyp forceps** and **nasal scissors** to fit up the nose.

Killian nasal speculums also come in a wide range of sizes and are obviously inserted into the nostril to gain access.

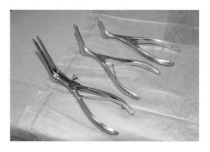

Killian nasal speculums.

42 Sutures

Matt Stephenson and Cheryl Funnell

> **Video** | **16 min 5 s**
> Cheryl Funnell, Lead Practitioner, General and
> Emergency Team and Registered Nurse,
> and Richard Harvey, Surgical Teaching Fellow
> Conquest Hospital, Hastings and Royal Sussex
> County Hospital, Brighton

Introduction

There is a bewildering array of sutures and, because there are different manufacturers, there are different commonly used names for essentially the same sutures. In general, it's acceptable to use the trade name of a suture in exams, as long as you know what it is and why you'd use it. You're also more likely to get a blank look from your scrub person if you ask for Polyglactin 910, rather than Vicryl.

Two of the commoner suture manufacturers are **Ethicon**™ and **Covidien**™. Your hospital may stock sutures from both suppliers, and there will be therefore a different

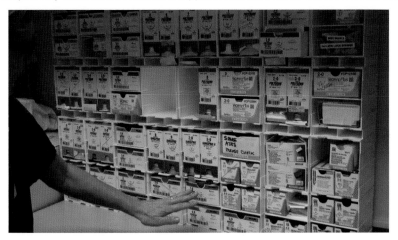

The average suture stack.

How to Operate: for MRCS Candidates and Surgical Trainees, First Edition. M. Stephenson. © 2011 John Wiley & Sons, Ltd.
Published 2011 by John Wiley & Sons, Ltd.

trade name for each supplier for what is, more or less, the same suture, making it very frustrating to learn them all. We'll discuss the common attributes of sutures that you need to be aware of to help you choose which one to use and then some examples of commonly used sutures.

If you really want to get into sutures though, there are many other characteristics to be aware of, which aren't covered here, like breaking strength (limit of tensile strength), capillarity (extent to which fluid is absorbed up its length), knot-pull tensile strength (tensile strength after knot tied), fluid absorption (amount of fluid absorbed after immersion), natural or synthetic etc. In the video we've also briefly touched on diathermy, various lotions and potions commonly used in theatre and some issues of theatre safety.

Absorbable versus non-absorbable

In a vascular anastomosis of Dacron graft to aorta, the join is never going to heal in the way a bowel anastomosis will. The suture must be as strong 20 years down the line as it is the day you put it in, so you need a **non-absorbable suture**. The same goes for hernia meshes. However, if what you're stitching together is eventually going to heal up, a bowel anastomosis, the linea alba, the fascia lata etc., you can use an **absorbable suture**, so that there won't forever be a foreign body there, to act as a nidus for infection for instance. Some tissues take longer to heal and therefore you will want to use suture material that dissolves over a longer time period.

Monofilament versus braided (polyfilament)

Ideally all sutures would be **monofilament** as there are fewer microscopic grooves and hiding places for organisms to fester and cause an infection. However, monofilament sutures have two significant disadvantages, firstly, they tend to have more **memory** (they keep recoiling to their awkward shape even if you stretch them out) and, secondly, they are **less strong**.

Size (thickness)

Whoever came up with the sizing system for suture thickness should be ashamed of him/herself. It is of course a throw-back to when sutures were much thicker. Originally they were numbered 1–6, 1 being the thinnest available, 6 the fattest. However, with great advances in suture manufacturing and materials technology, thinner sutures could be used instead with equivalent strength (and less foreign body). So they started numbering back to 0 and then 2–0, 3–0, 4–0 etc. down to 11–0, which is like trying to suture with a spider web, and only used in ophthalmic surgery. In general, it's rare now to use a suture thicker than a 1.

Needle type

Some of your more mature theatre sisters will tell you how they used to have to thread the suture through a hole in the needle. Of course this has been superseded by sutures that are attached to the needle already (using a process called swaging). The former were necessarily more traumatic as there would be a tiny bulge at the site where the needle had been threaded. The latter are described as **atraumatic** needles. There are a variety of **shapes** of needles and they also vary in the **geometry** of the point. Shapes include straight, 1/4 circle, 3/8 circle, 1/2 circle, 5/8 circle, J-shape, and can be selected mainly based on the space you have available to put the stitch in. A J-shaped needle is ideal, for instance, in getting down a deep, dark laparoscopic port hole for instance. Point geometry variations include:

Round body—which smoothly tapers to the point—a commonly used standard needle. They make the smallest possible hole in the tissue, good for anastomoses but not really strong enough for tough skin.

Cutting—triangular needle body with extra sharp cutting edge on the inside (i.e. on the side of the wound edge) for tougher tissues.

Reverse cutting—again for tougher tissues but having the cutting edge on the outside, that is not the side of the wound edge which means there's less likelihood of the needle cutting out through the tissue edge.

Tapercut—a cutting needle body that also tapers to a diameter not exceeding that of the suture (ideally) thus attempting to combine the powers of both the round body and cutting needle.

Blunt—no sharp point but can still be passed through some tissues like in mass closure of the abdomen with less risk of pranging bowel or your fingers.

Specific examples

The commonest absorbable sutures you're likely to come across in most surgical practice are **Vicryl** or **Polysorb** (roughly equivalent). They can be used for general ligating and transfixing of vessels or chunks of tissue, or closing layers of tissue in most cases. The average thickness is 2–0. So if in doubt in your exam, the answer is probably 2–0 Vicryl. For thicker leashes of tissue or bigger vessels, use a thicker thread like 0 Vicryl. It's important to choose an appropriate thickness of thread for the tissue you're ligating. You wouldn't tie a boat to a dock with a fishing line just as you wouldn't use a rope to go fishing. They can be used for closing skin too, although, because skin heals quickly, many people prefer to use **Vicryl Rapide**, or **Monocryl** or **Caprosyn** (roughly equivalent), to minimise the time foreign material is in the wound. Also you wouldn't want to use Vicryl or Polysorb to close tissue that will take several weeks to heal—the linea alba after a laparotomy for instance. Here, **PDS** or **Maxon** (roughly equivalent) will do the job.

The main non-absorbable sutures in common use are **Prolene** or **Surgipro** (roughly equivalent) which are biologically inert and have good strength—use them for vascular anastomoses and hernia repairs. Again, 2–0 is the average, for instance for a hernia repair, or for a large vascular anastomosis like the aorta to a graft, whereas 7–0 would be used for a radiocephalic fistula. **Nylon** sutures tend to be used mainly for interrupted sutures when closing skin but are also useful for incisional or paraumbilical hernias where you want the tissue to be held together for as long as possible to give it time to heal. **Silk** sutures have disadvantages, mainly because they're braided and can cause a biological reaction in the tissue. They are generally reserved for stitching in the drain, marking a specimen or practising tying knots.

Commonly used sutures with some of their important characteristics

	Ethicon name	Covidien name	Half-life and complete absorption	Mono or braided	Examples of use
Absorbable	PDS (polydioxanone)	Maxon (polytrimethylene carbonate)	T½: 21 A: 180	Mono	Mass closure
	Monocryl (poliglecaprone 25)	Caprosyn (polyglytone 6211)	T½: 5–7 A: 21	Mono	Subcuticular
	Vicryl (Polyglactin 910)	Polysorb (Lactomer copolymer)	T½: 14–21 A: 56–70	Braided	Very versatile, commonly used suture
	Vicryl rapide (polyglactin 910)		T½: 5 A: 42	Braided	Subcuticular
Non-absorbable	Prolene (polypropylene)	Surgipro (polypropylene)	N/A	Mono	Vascular anastomoses, hernia repairs
	Ethilon (nylon)	Monosof (nylon)	N/A	Mono	Skin stitches
	Permahand silk (silk)	Sofsilk (silk)	N/A	Braided	Drain stitches

T ½, half-life in days; A, complete absorption in days, N/A, not applicable.

43 Patient Safety and the WHO Surgical Checklist

Matt Stephenson and Christopher M Butler

Introduction

A relatively new, hot topic in surgery is **patient safety**. But what does that mean exactly? The true magnitude of adverse events for patients during their time in contact with healthcare services was underappreciated until the 1990s. Statistics like '1 in 10 patients affected by an adverse event' during their inpatient stay raised a few eyebrows. In 2007 in England and Wales, a whopping 129 419 incidents relating to surgical specialties were reported to the **National Learning and Reporting Service** (a branch of the NPSA, see later)—including 271 deaths—and that's just the ones that were reported (bear in mind that reporting adverse events is now more than ever considered a crucial part of our duties as doctors). All sorts of factors impact on errors in patient care, from simple human errors to complex systemic failures. This is a growing discipline of healthcare science. But what is most relevant to our practice as surgeons now?

The **National Patient Safety Agency** (**NPSA**) is charged with the responsibility for patient safety within the NHS and a check of their website (www.npsa.nhs.uk) will reveal a wide variety of guidelines for aspects of surgical and anaesthetic care, from alerts about the use of throat packs to avoiding wrong-side surgery for burr holes. Make yourself aware of these guidelines and advice—they're there for a reason—serious problems have happened in the past, which have resulted in harm to patients. There's only one thing better than learning from your own mistakes, and that's learning from someone else's.

What's the worst thing that could happen to you in your career? Your patient's anastomosis breaks down? You get a complaint from a patient because they had to wait too long for their hip replacement? Your young road traffic accident victim didn't survive

How to Operate: for MRCS Candidates and Surgical Trainees, First Edition. M. Stephenson. © 2011 John Wiley & Sons, Ltd. Published 2011 by John Wiley & Sons, Ltd.

their serious injuries despite your heroic efforts? How about taking out the **wrong kidney**? Or getting your **patients mixed up** and stripping someone's long saphenous vein when you were supposed to be fixing their hernia? Or performing major elective vascular surgery, and realise too late that there's **no blood available** and they exsanguinate? In the first three, within reason there's probably nothing else you could have done. The latter examples are catastrophic, avoidable and violate the first rule of the Hippocratic Oath: **first, do no harm**.

The Patient Safety Checklist

In June 2008, the **World Health Organisation** launched a global initiative (as by no means is this problem peculiar to the UK) called **Safe Surgery Saves Lives**. At the core of this, is a **simple checklist**. The idea behind it is to partially ritualise the process of perioperative care to make certain that in every single case, the most significant errors are avoided. Some of these errors have been termed **'never events'**, in other words they should in no circumstances ever occur because they are avoidable and disastrous.

The checklist (see the copy reproduced here) comprises **three stages: sign in, time out and sign out**. One member of the theatre staff—and it can be anyone, including you—must read each of these steps out aloud to the team. They may vary slightly from hospital to hospital, but this is the blueprint.

Sign in

Before the patient is even induced, the first part of the checklist must be completed. **Firstly**, has the patient **confirmed his or her identity**, the **procedure** they're having and have they **signed the consent form**? Probably the most crucial step of all—and it's generally taken for granted by us as surgeons—is that the right patient will turn up on the operating table. But without this step, you are essentially entrusting your GMC registration to the quality of your hospital porters. **Secondly**, **is the site or side marked**? In *every* case, if the operation is planned on one side of the body, they *must* be marked preoperatively, with the patient awake and witnessing where you're marking them so they can correct you if you're wrong. It doesn't matter if it's the only foot that's gangrenous or the only groin with a massive lump poking out (which may reduce on lying down and muscle relaxation). **Thirdly**, **is the anaesthesia machine and medication check complete**? Yes, well, presumably that would be important but one doesn't want to trifle too much with what the anaesthetists do. **Fourthly**, does the patient have a **known allergy**? The importance of which speaks for itself. Put away your betadine if it turns out they're allergic to iodine. **Fifthly**, is there likely to be a **difficult airway or aspiration risk**? Should you have put a nasogastric tube into your bowel obstructed patient before

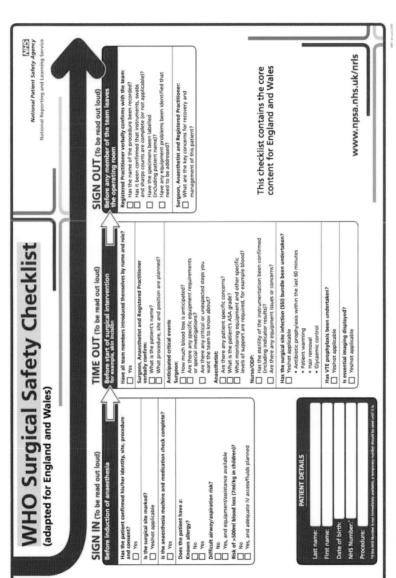

WHO Surgical Safety Checklist
(adapted for England and Wales)

National Patient Safety Agency
National Reporting and Learning Service

SIGN IN (To be read out loud)

Before induction of anaesthesia

Has the patient confirmed his/her identity, site, procedure and consent?
☐ Yes

Is the surgical site marked?
☐ Yes/not applicable

Is the anaesthesia machine and medication check complete?
☐ Yes

Does the patient have a:

Known allergy?
☐ No
☐ Yes

Difficult airway/aspiration risk?
☐ No
☐ Yes, and equipment/assistance available

Risk of >500ml blood loss (7ml/kg in children)?
☐ No
☐ Yes, and adequate IV access/fluids planned

PATIENT DETAILS

Last name:

First name:

Date of birth:

NHS Number:

Procedure:

TIME OUT (To be read out loud)

Before start of surgical intervention
for example, skin incision

Have all team members introduced themselves by name and role?
☐ Yes

Surgeon, Anaesthetist and Registered Practitioner verbally confirms:
☐ What is the patient's name?
☐ What procedure, site and position are planned?

Anticipated critical events

Surgeon:
☐ How much blood loss is anticipated?
☐ Are there any specific equipment requirements or special investigations?
☐ Are there any critical or unexpected steps you want the team to know about?

Anaesthetist:
☐ Are there any patient specific concerns?
☐ What is the patient's ASA grade?
☐ What monitoring equipment and other specific levels of support are required, for example blood?

Nurse/ODP:
☐ Has the sterility of the instrumentation been confirmed (including indicator results)?
☐ Are there any equipment issues or concerns?

Has the surgical site infection (SSI) bundle been undertaken?
☐ Yes/not applicable
  • Antibiotic prophylaxis within the last 60 minutes
  • Patient warming
  • Hair removal
  • Glycaemic control

Has VTE prophylaxis been undertaken?
☐ Yes/not applicable

Is essential imaging displayed?
☐ Yes/not applicable

SIGN OUT (To be read out loud)

Before any member of the team leaves the operating room

Registered Practitioner verbally confirms with the team:
☐ Has the name of the procedure been recorded?
☐ Has it been confirmed that instruments, swabs and sharps counts are complete (or not applicable)?
☐ Have the specimens been labelled (including patient name)?
☐ Have any equipment problems been identified that need to be addressed?

Surgeon, Anaesthetist and Registered Practitioner:
☐ What are the key concerns for recovery and management of this patient?

This checklist contains the core content for England and Wales

www.npsa.nhs.uk/nrls

THIS CHECKLIST IS NOT INTENDED TO BE COMPREHENSIVE. ADDITIONS AND MODIFICATIONS TO FIT LOCAL PRACTICE ARE ENCOURAGED.

Patient Safety and the WHO Surgical Checklist | **233**

induction? **Sixthly**, is the risk of **blood loss** likely to be **greater than 500 ml** (or in a **child 7 ml/kg**)? In which case make sure blood resources are available to you if necessary.

Time out

The patient is now asleep and on the table. The theatre team reassembles and **introduces themselves by name and role**. Obviously this is particularly important if you're new to the theatre, but even in theatres with consistent staff and the consultant's been there for 30 years, think about how often there's an agency nurse or a new medical student. One infamous case of a 'wrong side' nephrectomy occurred despite the medical student noticing they were about to operate on the wrong side and flagging it up—she was ignored. The concept of **flattened hierarchy** is that no longer should anyone feel they're not important enough to raise a concern. The HCA should be able to tell the consultant she's noticed the patient has a pacemaker and that therefore monopolar diathermy is contraindicated, for instance. By getting everyone's names and roles clear at the start, **communication** between the team can then flow much better.

You must then check again—what is the **patient's name**, what **procedure** are you planning, on **which side**, and what **position** do you want the patient in? It may sound far fetched but cases have occurred when the patient who came into the anaesthetic room is not the one who comes on to the operating table. Imagine you are on call and this is the emergency list. Your patient was in the anaesthetic room and you were called off to A and E for an emergency. You return to theatre half an hour later to drain said patient's abscess, only in the time you were gone an urgent testicular torsion took precedence over your patient who's been returned to the ward. It has happened! Don't rely on everyone else to prevent your mistakes.

As doctors we don't tend to like protocols, but in some cases they can truly get you out of some very unpleasant situations. Put up with the fact that perhaps 99% of the time there are no hidden surprises, in order to safeguard that one patient, and you, from those odd freakish out-of-nowhere events that will have life changing consequences not only for your patient, but for you.

Next, you want to warn the team about any **critical events you anticipate**. This could range from needing a rigid sigmoidoscope to assess the rectal mucosa when draining a perianal abscess, to a crucial piece of equipment you might need should something go wrong. There is then the rather unfortunately phrased: 'Are there any **critical or unexpected steps** you want the team to know about?' It doesn't mean 'do you expect there to be any unexpected steps', that would indeed make no sense, it means are there any steps that you know might happen but the team weren't expecting (however, this question invariably invokes incomprehension and derision from theatre staff every single time it's mentioned)? How much **blood loss** are you anticipating? Of course it may be difficult to say, but you're best placed to make an educated guess. There are also some questions for the anaesthetist regarding their concerns and their ASA grade etc., and also for the scrub person.

If you haven't heard of the **Surgical Site Infection Bundle**, here it is. It comprises four aspects of care that have an evidence base to reduce the risk of surgical site infection. Quite why it's called a bundle is anybody's guess.

1 Has **hair removal** been performed adequately? Ideally it should be avoided altogether but where necessary it should be done with clippers, not razors, and with minimal disruption of the skin as possible, and close to the time of surgery.

2 If **antibiotics** are indicated (always for instance when bowel may be opened, including **always** before an appendicectomy) have they been given within 60 minutes prior to the operation?

3 Has the patient's **blood glucose** been adequately normalised?

4 Has the patient's **temperature** been adequately normalised?

The morbidity from **venous thromboembolism** is very significant to us all in our surgical practice. All patients must be **assessed** for their need for low molecular weight heparin and intraoperative pneumatic calf compression or at least thromboembolic deterrent stockings (TEDS). Finally, are the relevant **images** up on the computer screen or X-ray box? If you need to see a mammogram to help guide you in your wide local excision, you don't want an added 10 minutes of anaesthetic time whilst someone runs around the ward trying to find it.

Sign out

Once the procedure has been completed, there is a third and final step to the process. The **name of the procedure** needs to be clearly stated (it often seems strange, when you've been slaving away at a laparotomy for the last 2 hours, how often no one else in the theatre actually knows quite what you've been doing (often least of all the anaesthetist)). This enables safe handover to the recovery staff and recording of the procedure in the log. The scrub person **must confirm that the final count of swabs, needles and instruments are correct** (by the way, when they tell you this, don't just ignore it—thank them, it's also for your benefit— who do you think will be in court if a swab's left in the abdomen?). The **specimens** must be appropriately **labelled** and any **faulty equipment reported** and acted on. Finally, are there any **concerns for recovery** on the ward for the ongoing management of this patient? Do they, for instance, have palpable pulses at the end of the operation and would you want to know if they vanish?

Summary

The WHO surgical safety checklist is not a tick box exercise. OK, so it is in fact exactly a tick box exercise, but, for it to have value, it must be much more than that. It is not simply the observance of these steps in order to get through them quickly to satisfy sister; much more important is the **spirit** in which the checklist is handled. It is there for **your benefit** as much as anyone else's. It is there to prevent a once in a career event that could ruin your patient's life, and yours. It's there to help mitigate against our natural **human tendency to err**, even if we're so superhuman we only err once every few decades. What's more, there is an evidence base to it. Despite all of that, you will find that surgeons are split about its usefulness, in common with pretty much anything else 'new' that's ever been introduced to an established system, be it Ignez Semmelweiss's attempts to introduce hand washing in the 1840s or laparoscopic surgery in the 1970s. Get used to it, embrace it, it's here to stay.

44 Theatre Etiquette

Matt Stephenson and Ginny Bowbrick

Introduction

Theatre is a unique environment and one in which as a surgeon you will want to be most comfortable in. Sometimes on entering a new theatre, you find yourself entering a peculiar world filled with fragile egos, ambitious career climbers, clandestine political wrangling and complex power struggles. Patients also have operations there. For that reason, learning to grease your way through this often complicated domain is very important.

You might broadly divide the rules you should observe into **Before**, **During** and **After** the operation. It is in general just common sense.

Before the operation

Few things are more like a red rag to a bull for a consultant than turning up to his list without doing a bit of **groundwork beforehand**. Not going to **see the patient** before the operation, or at least having a good **read of the notes** and **review of the imaging** if applicable, is asking for trouble and no chance of being allowed to operate on that particular patient. It is a good idea to bring up any relevant imaging such as CT scans or arteriograms on the theatre computer and this can also turn into an impromptu teaching session with the boss while waiting for the patient to be anaesthetised. But it's not enough to know the patient; you need to have some idea of **what the operation is about** too. Read about and watch the video the night

before if you know what's on the next list. The sooner you show that you know and understand the operation, the sooner you'll be allowed to do it yourself.

It's a favourite pastime of all surgeons to conveniently forget that their **knowledge of anatomy** probably wasn't very good at your stage of training either, but still scoff and bemoan the demise in undergraduate anatomy education if you can't recall some obscure anatomical fact. In fairness, there is probably some truth in this—anatomy has taken a battering in many undergraduate courses. Make sure you've opened an anatomy textbook and/or atlas before the operation so that you can at least guess the answer to any questions fired at you.

If it's your first time in a particular theatre and you're not familiar with the theatre

How to Operate: for MRCS Candidates and Surgical Trainees, First Edition. M. Stephenson. © 2011 John Wiley & Sons, Ltd. Published 2011 by John Wiley & Sons, Ltd.

staff—**introduce yourself** before the list starts. With a theatre sister not known for her friendliness to new intruders, having a little one-to-one time in theatre will make it a lot more challenging for her to make your life more difficult. **Communication is key** to the successful running of a theatre list—if, for instance, you know of a change in circumstances that will affect the list, let the theatre staff know as soon as you can. **Respect the theatre staff**—they often have an extraordinary amount of knowledge and experience, which will often help you out in times of trouble. If left to operate without the boss, an experienced scrub nurse may for instance suggest instruments that the boss uses at different steps of the operation but if you have not made any effort to get to know them then they will not. Never underestimate the relationship between the long-standing theatre staff and your boss.

Dress appropriately. It's obvious what you should and shouldn't wear but it's surprising to see how many new students or trainees arrive in theatre with a big fringe hanging down from under their hat or bling jewellery dripping off their fingers. Some theatres have colour coded hats such as green for students and blue for qualified staff whether medical or nursing so it pays to ask first if this applies in each hospital you work in. Don't wear your identification badge dangling somewhere near your genitals where people can only look at it by making themselves feel uncomfortable. If you need to speak to someone in theatre, it's always best to get **changed into scrubs** and go inside rather than trying to talk through a crack in the doorway (although often very impractical). It's usually best to pass a message through the scrub person who can then speak to the operating surgeon at an appropriate time. **Never ever** wear someone else's clogs or you may end up with an irate and bare foot consultant hunting you down from theatre to theatre.

When watching an operation, make a big show of taking great care of **preserving the sterile field**—don't for instance walk between the scrub person's sterile trolley and the operating table. Avoid walking around the anaesthetic end of the table when scrubbed—remember all surgeons view anaesthetists as dirty.

You need to get the theatre staff on side. It is immeasurably important. **Make yourself useful** and show you're happy to muck in with whatever needs to be done and that you have no airs and graces about doing so. If the phone is ringing in theatre—answer it. If there's a dirty swab dropped on the floor—pick it up. When the patient is transferred—help. If there are no snacks or sugary treats in the preparation room—buy some. Be ready to catheterise the male or female patients if required.

Leave your bleep wherever it's supposed to be left (often this is at the front desk of theatres) or, if you can, hand it to a colleague to cover. **Return the favour**

for them another time. Don't screw your colleagues over. **Turn off your mobile phone**. Don't be shy about asking to scrub up. Obey the World Health Organisation **(WHO) checklist** (see *Patient Safety* Chapter 43), or instigate it yourself.

During the operation

Get to know your consultant's **glove and gown size** and open it for them before the case as well as for yourself. **Scrub thoroughly** in the usual way and always **scrub for slightly longer** than the next most senior person to you. Hold your hands together across your chest when walking from the sink towards the table, and maintain sterility at all times.

When assisting, look and **be attentive** but **don't grovel**. If and when it seems appropriate try and **ask appropriate questions** but don't be too talkative, unless that's the way your boss is. Suggestions and discussion of technique and steps in the operation are welcome—criticisms or saying how much better your last boss did something are not. Don't yawn and don't gossip with the other staff. Try to **blend in** with whatever the mood and ethos of that theatre seems to be. **Make yourself as useful as possible** when assisting. Try to anticipate what the operating surgeon is about to do next, which often takes a lot of practise as you may not yet know the next step, but if a knot's being tied for instance, you're likely to need to cut the suture soon, so have scissors ready.

But of course, you don't want to be assisting all your life. You want to **get your hands on the knife**. Your success in this depends on many things, not least the generosity, patience and self-confidence of your boss (perhaps the three most important characteristics to have in a trainer) and the relationship you develop with them. Make sure you **know the basics**: suture, tie knots, hold instruments etc. The Basic Surgical Skills course helps with this. Many bosses will judge whether you can do the operation on whether you can assist well, so get the basics right. Borrow instruments from theatre to practise with in the coffee room and practise tying knots—there is many a surgical trainee's bag or theatre coffee room chair leg with Vicryl ties hanging from them used to practice knot tying until smoothly performed.

If you're not getting much operating, **make it known** gently that you're very interested in getting your hands on such and such a case. Tell him or her you've assisted in X number of procedures before and demonstrate your knowledge of the steps, and hint at how hard you've been working on the wards. If this doesn't work, your options range from purposely finishing scrubbing before your boss and then standing on the operating side of the table, to snatching the knife out of his hand. The latter, in general, is not recommended. If all else fails talk to your Surgical Tutor about your predicament.

When the patient is **awake**, under local anaesthetic—the atmosphere in theatre is usually very different. Remember you are there purely for that patient. Their comfort should be the focus of everyone's attention. They should have someone available to talk to them (unless also sedated) all the way through. Take great care to remember all the way through the operation that the patient is awake and refrain from discussing your plans for the weekend or a recent mess party. In some theatres, a large sign is placed in a highly visible place to remind everyone—it can be easily forgotten. Ask the patient if they would like to listen to music during the procedure and if so listen to what they would like rather than your preference.

All consultants have their own way of doing things such as a preferred skin suture so if allowed to operate on one of their patients then it is only polite to do what they prefer otherwise you will find yourself no longer operating on their patients, and rest assured the theatre scrub nurse will tell them if you digress. If you also always do it your consultant's way whilst you're working for them, for example doing all the dissection with a knife or scissors rather than the diathermy pencil, it also allows you to build up a wider range of skills by the end of your training. Eventually, you'll be able to decide the way you prefer to do it.

After the operation

You haven't finished the operation until you have helped **transfer the patient back** on to the bed. **Clean up** any detritus on the floor or around the operating trolley—**make yourself useful**. Offer to make the boss a coffee or take the op notes when written through to recovery—an all-day list requires a lot of concentration and is tiring, so these things will help to enhance your relationship with your boss.

It is mandatory to **go and see your patient** afterwards and let him or her know how it went. Sometimes at the end of a late list, that's very difficult to do, especially if it's anticipated they'll take a long time to wake up. Make sure that at least the nursing staff or on call surgeon are well informed from your op note. Make the **op note as clear as possible** with your postoperative instructions (see *How to Write the Operation Note* Chapter 45). **Thank everyone** in theatre, especially if you've delayed the list because you were being trained. If you performed the operation try to have a **debrief** with your trainer on what you did well and not so well, preferably in the format of a **Procedure-Based Assessment (PBA)**. Record the operation in your **logbook**.

45 How to Write the Operation Note

Matt Stephenson and Petra Marsh

Writing the operation note is one of those things no one ever shows you how to do. In truth, it's not difficult and you basically just write down what you did. But there are a few simple things to remember to include and a commonly used standard format adopted by many surgeons for most operations.

You want your operation note to be **easily found** in the notes, to **accurately answer** any questions a nurse or doctor might have when looking after your patient on their first postoperative night and contain **all the useful information** that might be sought 10 years down the line. The more experienced you become and the more hospitals you travel around, and then back to years later, the more you come across your own operative record written years back—you can then judge your own work retrospectively.

It's obvious of course, but begin by putting the **patient details** at the top of the page—**name**, **hospital number** and **date of birth** as a minimum. Put the **date** in the left margin and the **time** of the operation—not so essential for elective cases but for emergency ones it's more important. Some people like to write the **start time** (knife to skin) and the **end time** (closed up) with an arrow between the two; it's often helpful to know how long the operation took.

So on to the operation note itself. What **colour** do you write it in? Well you will doubtlessly have heard innumerable times that you mustn't write in the notes in **red ink**. This dates back to **preancient times** when photocopiers struggled to copy red ink in the event that your notes might be requested by the coroner or similar. Well if you can find a photocopier these days that can't photocopy red ink, hats off to you. The idea of using red ink is that when you're in a hurry leafing through vast volumes of notes, 95% of which are taken up by **completely superfluous paperwork** you can more rapidly identify the important operation note. However, if your Trust condemns such practice, obviously one must submit and write it in black.

In some hospitals it's normal practice to **type** all operative notes. This is particularly helpful if your handwriting isn't up

How to Operate: for MRCS Candidates and Surgical Trainees, First Edition. M. Stephenson. © 2011 John Wiley & Sons, Ltd. Published 2011 by John Wiley & Sons, Ltd.

South Forest NHS Trust
South River Hospital

Patient Name	Tom Thumb		
Hosp No.	100546783		
Date of birth	12/03/1985		

Date	21/11/2010	Surgeon	T Best
Elective/emergency	emergency	Assistant	F Tryer
Consultant	Mr N Bottom	Anaesthetist	A Gassman
		Type of anaesthetic	GA

VTE prophylaxis	LMW heparin 20/11/10	WHO Safe surgery checklist	✓
	20.00	Position	supine
	TEDS	Start	14.00
Antibiotic prophylaxis	amoxicillin	Finish	14.35
	gentamicin		

Indication for surgery	pain & tenderness Mc Burney's point
Operation	Open appendicectomy
Operative Diagnosis	acute appendicitis
Operative Codes	E2341

Incision	Lanz, muscle-splitting
Findings	acutely inflamed appendix, no free peritoneal fluid or pus
	No fluid in pelvis
Procedure	Mesoappendix divided between clamps, ligated using 2/0 absorbable ties
	Appendix base crushed & clamp applied distally. 0 absorbable tie to base.
	Appendix excised leaving short stump and sent for histology
Closure	peritoneum closed under direct vision 2/0 absorbable continuous suture
	Then layered closure:
	TA & IO closed with loose apposition suture
	EO continuous closure 2/0 absorbable suture

Local anaesthetic	20ml 0.5% bupivacaine block to wound
Drains	none
Samples	appendix specimen to histopathology

Postoperative Instructions

Routine postoperative observations
Start eating and drinking as tolerated
2 more doses of antibiotics
LMW heparin and TEDS as prescribed

Example of an operation note.

to scratch. The only caveat to this is—make sure it is typed straight away—not dictated onto tape to be typed the next day. If your patient has a problem in the middle of the night and the team looking after him don't have the op note to find out what went on in theatre you'll be in big trouble.

At the top of the page write:

OPERATION NOTE (if it's not preprinted)

And below this, the name of the operation, for instance:

RIGHT INGUINAL HERNIA REPAIR

Then put:

Surgeon: YOUR NAME
Assistant: SOMEONE ELSE'S NAME

Then the form of **anaesthesia** used, **who** did it, if any **antibiotics** were given and what **venous thromboembolism prophylaxis** measures were taken. For some situations it's also worth writing down the patient's ASA.

G.A. + ILIOINGUINAL NERVE BLOCK: DR. GAS

You should then say whether this was an **elective** case or an **emergency** case done on the CEPOD list; sometimes it's obvious but occasionally it's not and that can be useful in the future and also helps the clinical coders (the people that break down all hospital episodes into codes, and codes mean prizes, for the hospital at least). In some hospitals you even have to look up the code yourself.

Did you know why the emergency list is called a **CEPOD** list by the way? In the olden days emergencies would go to theatre as and when, tacked onto the end of elective lists (as they still do sometimes) or carry through into the middle of the night. In 1982 there was a study, **Confidential Enquiry into Peri Operative Deaths**, looking at outcomes from surgery and anaesthesia dependent on various factors including when it was performed. One of the outcomes was that it was best not to do non-life- or limb-threatening surgery in the middle of the night and recommendations were made to create dedicated theatre space during the day to accommodate emergencies. This enquiry was the precursor to the formation of the National Confidential Enquiry into Patient Outcome and Death (NCEPOD), which has looked into many other clinical governance issues. We digress. So simply state:

EMERGENCY (CEPOD list)

Then write the **indication** for the surgery, although this isn't always necessary as it's often self evident in why you're doing the operation, but you might do a Hartmann's procedure for instance either because of bowel obstruction or perforation.

Indication: INCARCERATED INGUINAL HERNIA

So now to the nitty gritty of it. For most operations you can follow the same formula: **Incision**, **Findings**, **Procedure**,

Closure, usually abbreviated to I, F, P and C.

I: Right groin crease

Then tell them the punchline straight away, **what did you find**? After going through the skin, everybody gets to the hernia in roughly the same way so you don't have to repeat every obvious step about going through fat, fascia etc. **Diagrams** can be really useful, they don't have to be complex but when trying to explain, for instance, what vessel you anastomosed onto what or what the configuration of the fracture and your plates and screws were, a picture tells a thousand words.

F: Incarcerated indirect inguinal hernia
  Sac containing viable omentum, no bowel
  No direct hernia

So **what did you do** about it?

P: Sac dissected and opened
  Cord structures identified and preserved
  Sac contents inspected and returned to abdomen
  Sac transfixed and divided
  Polypropylene mesh shaped and sutured in place
  Haemostasis

Include any biopsies or microbiology samples taken. And then how did you **close the wound** and did you put in any more local anaesthetic?

C: External oblique—Vicryl 2–0 continuous
  Fat/superficial fascia—Vicryl 2–0 interrupted

Skin—Subcuticular continuous monocryl 3–0
Opsite dressing to skin

Finally, what are your **postoperative instructions**. It's really important to be as clear on this as possible. If you don't know when the drain should come out or when the patient should start mobilising on their fixed fracture how will anyone else? Were there pulses in the affected limb at the end of the operation? Can they eat and drink?

Post op: Can eat and drink when desires
  Routine ward observations
  Aim for home tomorrow after review

Make sure that the **drug chart** has everything necessary prescribed—do they need antibiotic cover, for how many days and what is the indication? Do they need low molecular weight heparin DVT prophylaxis? What analgesia is pre-scribed? If the patient is a day case it's usually best to write the **discharge letter** along with a prescription for any medications to take away at the same time as the op note just to save time.

Of course, not all operations conform to this system and you can adapt it as much as you see fit as long as it's still clear. Just make sure you've included all the import-ant things. It's a general rule of thumb when writing any notes that you write as much detail as you would want to have at your disposal in the unfortunate scenario of having to explain something to the coroner. So for instance, if you changed the prearranged plan midway through an operation because of unforeseen circumstances and called your boss to discuss it—say so. If you carefully checked there was no bleeding at the end of the operation put it in.

Your operation is not over of course until you've helped **transfer** the patient back on to their bed. Then write the note. It's usually best, especially if it's been a long case, to leave the theatre for a few moments and **sit down** quietly in the coffee room to write all this out. Perching the notes on the edge of the catheter trolley whilst the anaesthetist's shouting at the patient to wake up and the floor's being mopped around you is not conducive to good note writing. Make sure that the op note is **filed in the right place** in the notes not just tucked in the front to get lost, and then take the notes round to recovery.

46 Consent

Matt Stephenson

It is well established that, as a general rule, the performance of a medical operation upon a person without his or her consent is unlawful, as constituting both the crime of battery and the tort of trespass to the person
Lord Goff 1990

Introduction

Consenting the patient means that irritating step of getting them to sign that yellow form before the porters take them down to theatre, doesn't it? Well unfortunately that's how it's often interpreted, and practised. Consent to many may sound like a boring dry subject, but if you want to be a surgeon, you'd better get interested in it, and fully understand it. If you don't, a career's worth of disgruntled patients, lawsuits, and even (theoretically) a spell in one of Her Majesty's prisons, awaits you. This by no means will be a comprehensive review of consent—it would take up several tomes – this is a brief whistle stop tour.

Issues of consent for surgical procedures fall into two broad categories: those patients who **can consent for themselves**, and **those who can't**. In most of your practice, unless you're destined to be a neonatal paediatric surgeon, it's likely that the majority of your patients fall into the former group, and the distinguishing feature of the two groups is whether the patient has the mental capacity to make a decision.

Assessment of capacity

To decide which group your patient falls into, you need to decide if they have capacity to make decisions about their treatment. The first principle is that you **assume all patients over the age of 16 to have the required capacity** unless shown otherwise.

According to the **Mental Capacity Act (MCA) 2005**, a patient will not have capacity if he or she is unable to do one or more of the following:

1 **Understand** the information relevant to the decision
2 **Retain** that information
3 **Weigh up** the **pros and cons** related to the decision
4 **Communicate** the decision

Often, the above is not completely clear cut and everyone, including the courts, accept this. What is important is that you make reasonable decisions and **document clearly** in the notes anything that may seem contentious and how you've come to your conclusion. Furthermore, a patient may have the capacity to make decisions about one thing, but not another, or this may vary over time.

Patients with capacity

Assessment of capacity is just the first step for this group, there are two other vital ingredients to obtaining consent. The three components are:

1 The patient has **capacity** (see above)
2 The patient is **fully informed** about the procedure
3 The consent is **voluntary**

In other words, it's no good getting a perfectly competent, intelligent patient to consent to a procedure unless you have fully informed them of the nature of the procedure, the pros and cons and the alternatives. Equally, consent isn't valid if you've twisted their arm because you really wanted to do their operation, or you misrepresent the value of an alternative option or the patient is being bullied into it by a caring relative.

This second point is a bit sticky—just how much do you tell the patient about the risks of a procedure? For this we must look to some **English case law**. You may have heard of the **Bolam (and Bolitho) tests**. As Mr Justice McNair put it in Bolam in 1957:

I myself would prefer to put it this way, that he is not guilty of negligence if he has acted in accordance with a practice accepted as proper by a responsible body of medical men skilled in that particular art. I do not think there is much difference in sense. It is just a different way of expressing the same thought. Putting it the other way round, a man is not negligent, if he is acting in accordance with such a practice, merely because there is a body of opinion who would take a contrary view. At the same time, that does not mean that a medical man can obstinately and pig-headedly carry on with some old technique if it has been proved to be contrary to what is really substantially the whole of informed medical opinion. Otherwise you might get men today saying: 'I do not believe in anaesthetics. I do not believe in antiseptics. I am going to continue to do my surgery in the way it was done in the eighteenth century.' That clearly would be wrong.

This applied to consent in that a doctor would be expected to tell his patient about whatever risks a responsible body of doctors would tell their patients in the same circumstances.

In other words, if Doctor X never warned his hernia repair patients about the risk of chronic groin pain and a patient sues Doctor X because he didn't warn him, Dr X could get away with it if he could find a group of his mates who wouldn't have warned the patient in those circumstances either, *providing* that those mates held a view that was capable of withstanding logical analysis; a decision which would ultimately fall to be made by the Court.

This dominated the legal scene for a long time—and amounted to telling the patient about all of the common potential risks—but the crucial factor has been:

how common does a risk have to be to tell the patient? In the case of **Sidaway v Bethlem Royal Hospital** (1985), the claimant failed in her lawsuit against her neurosurgeon for not telling her about the 1% risk of paraplegia (which she unfortunately developed) during a cervical cord decompression. The court felt that the surgeon was not under a duty to warn the patient about remote side effects, they felt a risk of 10% was a reasonable cut off. In the case of **Pearce v United Bristol** (1999), the pregnant complainant was overdue by about 2 weeks and requested an induction or caesarean section. She was advised by her consultant to proceed with a natural delivery but this resulted in a stillbirth. She lost her case because the risk of proceeding with a natural birth was only in the order of 0.1–0.2% but the court did contend that doctors should **err on the side of generosity** in giving information to their patients.

Importantly, in the Pearce case, the Court found that if there was a significant risk which would affect the judgement of **a reasonable patient**, then in the normal course it is the responsibility of a doctor to inform the patient of that significant risk so that the patient can determine for him or herself as to what course s/he should adopt. However, this should only be done if the doctor believes that the disclosure of such information would not cause the patient significant harm or distress—the 'therapeutic privilege'.

The next big case to challenge the received wisdom of risk was **Chester v Afshar** (2004). Mrs Chester suffered neurological injury following neurosurgical intervention for her lower back and claimed to have never been warned about it, the risk being in the order of 1–2%. She won. A precedent had been set in which serious complications, even if they were unlikely, should be raised with the patient.

As if that didn't make it complicated enough, there was then the case of **Birch v UCL Hospital** (2008). Mrs Birch was admitted with a third nerve palsy and underwent a diagnostic angiogram to look for a cerebral aneurysm. She was appropriately counselled about the risks of the angiogram. She suffered a stroke, sued the hospital, and won—why? Because she wasn't told about the **alternatives**, and the pros and cons of the alternatives (and in particular an MRI which would not have had the risk of a stroke) so she was found to have been denied an opportunity to properly weigh the comparative risks and benefits of competing procedures.

So there has been a paradigm shift away from warning patients about risks that seem **reasonable to the doctor** (or body of doctors), to warning the patient about risks that would seem **reasonable to the patient**. In other words, a 0.5% risk of causing ischaemic orchitis following a primary inguinal hernia repair may not seem too troubling to you as the surgeon, but if you were the patient, you may have wanted to know. What's more—have you told your patient that whilst you can offer an open inguinal hernia repair, Mr X down the road could do it laparoscopically (and all that that might entail)?

In short—consent, even for a patient with capacity, can be very, very thorny. But in general you are far safer by telling the patient more, rather than less, even if the risk is small. And by the way, what if you don't actually write down on the consent form or in the notes that you've warned the patient that the varicose veins might come back? Who do you think the civil courts are going to believe—you or the patient? Sorry, but it will be the patient almost all of the time. Remember civil courts need only prove, on the 'balance of probabilities' (not 'beyond all reasonable doubt' as in criminal courts) and who will the court consider is more likely to remember what you said on that day 3 years ago when you saw the patient in day surgery? The patient who's only had one operation in her life and for whom it was a major event, or you, who's done hundreds of operations since then and can't even remember her name?

So essentially, it's not about getting that patient to scribble a mark on a yellow form—it's a matter of confirming they have capacity to make that decision, ensuring they are fully informed of the procedure and all it entails including the alternatives and finally letting them think and cogitate on it. It is not therefore best left until the day of surgery unless in emergency situations—it's far better done in the outpatient clinic. The scribbling on the 'form' is merely evidence that you said

what you did, when you did—it is not 'consent'.

Patients without capacity

But what about patients who you think don't have capacity to make decisions? The **Mental Capacity Act (MCA) 2005**, which came in to force in October 2007, pulled together much of the *ad hoc* case law that had accumulated over the years. It was designed to codify the underlying principles to protect patients who lack capacity. Let's say, for instance, a man with Down's syndrome with associated severe learning disabilities comes to see you in clinic—he has an inguinal hernia (this isn't an emergency). The patient has no living relatives and no other legally recognised directive. In the past, if the doctor felt it was in the best interests of the patient to have his hernia repaired, he would proceed.

So what should you do now? Firstly, is it possible that the patient **may regain his capacity** and you must consider if the decision for treatment is **delayable** until then? If so you should wait, but this usually isn't the case. Secondly, you must **enable the patient** as much as possible in taking part in the decision-making process—even if you can't get a full and clear idea of what they would want, the little information you can still glean is useful. Thirdly, you must consider any **premorbid wishes expressed**—either verbally or written in for instance an **advance directive** (a legally recognised statement made by the patient when he/she has capacity, to be invoked if he/she loses capacity) or if the patient has appointed a **lasting power of attorney** (someone who the patient appointed when they had capacity, to take on such decisions in the event that they lose capacity, it replaced the **enduring power of attorney**). Fourthly, you must take the views of those closest to the **patient** (even if not appointed as lasting powers of attorney)—usually the family, but also healthcare professionals. Normally, this is sufficient to form a decision, but that decision to treat must be a reasonable one and made only after, and on the basis of, this holistic assessment of the patient's interests. It must be written in the notes in full with a thorough explanation of why and how the decision was reached. There is usually a special form in your hospital to fill in too. This should be enough to make a safe, considered decision in the best interests of the patient and keep you out of trouble.

But what happens if the patient has no family? They live in a nursing home and all their friends and family are dead. They have no advance directive and there's no lasting power of attorney. They are unbefriended. Meet the **Independent Mental Capacity Advocate (IMCA)**. These are non-medical individuals who you must get in contact with in these circumstances; your hospital will have a local IMCA service. They will arrange to meet with you to discuss the best interests of the patient, the IMCA representing what

one would hope to be the best interests of the patient. In other words, the paternalism of days gone has vanished—doctor does not necessarily know best. Ignoring this would be extremely unwise.

Special circumstances
Emergencies

In the emergency situation where the patient has capacity to make decisions, you can obviously proceed as you normally would, although the steps are bound to be quicker and you, the patient and the court would accept that time for cogitation would be limited. Worrying about being sued over this must not delay a vital operation. In emergencies, what needs to be done, gets done. For the patient without capacity to make decisions, which may be an unconscious patient or one with long-term lack of capacity, you must act in the patient's best interests and provide only that treatment which is necessary (until capacity can be re-established)—in true traditional paternalist style—and without further ado.

Paediatrics

In the 16–18-year-old category, patients can consent for procedures, but strictly they can't refuse them against medical advice if this would not be in their best interests. Such rare situations require great tact and care. In the rarest of situations, an application to court may be necessary. In the under 16 category, in general, patients are deemed to be children and their parents must consent for them and act in the child's best interests. However, the case of **Gillick v West Norfolk** (1985) in which a child was prescribed contraception without the knowledge of her mother set a precedent. If the minor is able to understand the information, in much the same way as an adult—they are deemed **'Gillick competent'**—that is they are treated as an adult and can consent as such. The decision is reached on a case by case basis and will require you to consider the mental, emotional and chronological age of the child, their ability to understand and their ability to appreciate the consequences of their decision.

Summary

- **All patients over the age of 16 have the capacity** to make decisions unless shown otherwise
- A patient must be able to **understand**, **retain** and **weigh up** the information and be able to **communicate** it
- In a patient with capacity, consent must be **fully informed** and **voluntary** to be legally recognised
- Inform patients of all the **common risks** and any **potentially serious risks**, even if the chances are small; err on the side of more, rather than less
- The **Mental Capacity Act 2005** changed the management of patients without capacity
- **Advance Directives** and **Lasting Power of Attorney** need to be considered in decision making in those without capacity
- If in doubt, appoint an **Independent Mental Capacity Advocate** (IMCA)
- In **emergencies**, if in doubt, act in what you see as the **best interests** of the patient
- Patients aged **16–18 can consent** to treatment but **can't refuse** it
- Patients **under 16 can consent** to treatment if they are **Gillick competent**

Index

Note: page numbers in *italics* refer to figures and tables

abdominal aortic aneurysm repair 60–7
  anastomosis 64–5
  back bleeding 63, 65
  blood pressure 65–6
  clamping 63
  closure 66
  common iliac artery 62, 63, 64
  duodenum location 61, 62
  femoral pulse 65, 66
  grafts 64, 65
  haemostasis 62, 66
  incision 60–1
  inferior mesenteric artery 63, 66
  inflammatory 66
  laparotomy 61
  left renal vein 62, 66
  'let the legs in 65–6
  lumbar arteries 63
  notes 66
  procedure 60–6
  sac
    closure 66
    location 61
    management 63, 64
  sutures 63, 64, 65, 66
abscess
  burst 21
  closure 20
  corrugated drain 22
  curetting of lining 22
  diabetic foot 20, 21
  diathermy 22
  dressing 23
  examination under anaesthesia 21

haemostatic pack 22–3
incision/drainage 20–3
  procedure 21–3
irrigation 22
ischiorectal 22
lactational of breast 167
microbiology swab 21, 22
occurrence 20
perianal 20–1
pilonidal sinus 206, 208
splenic 138
supralevator induration 21
adrenal gland 110, 111
advance directive 249–50
airway risk 232, 234
allergies, patient 232
Allis forceps 220
amputation *see below* knee amputation
anaesthesia
  abscess drainage 21
  carotid endarterectomy 75, 77
  femorodistal bypass 85
  split skin graft 9, 11
  wedge resection of toe 22
anaesthesia machine check 232
anal stenosis 194
anatomy, knowledge of 237
aneurysm
  endovascular repair 60
  see also abdominal aortic aneurysm repair
anterior tibial artery, femorodistal bypass 87
antibiotics 235
  prophylactic for splenectomised
    patients 139

How to Operate: for MRCS Candidates and Surgical Trainees, First Edition. M. Stephenson. © 2011 John Wiley & Sons, Ltd.
Published 2011 by John Wiley & Sons, Ltd.

anus, haemostatic pack 194–5
appendicectomy 34–9
    appendix location/delivery 36, 37–8
    closure 37
    dressings 37
    incision 34–5, 38
    McBurney's point 34
    mesoappendix ligation/division 36–7, 38
    notes 37–8
    obese patients 38
    peritoneal cavity washing 37
    peritoneum 35–6
    procedure 34–7
    retrocaecal appendix 38
    Rutherford—Morrison incision 38
    staples 37
    subhepatic appendix 38
    sutures 37
arteriovenous fistula 91
artery forceps 219–20
aspiration risk 232, 234
atherosclerotic disease 74
axilla, anatomy 172–3
axillary node clearance 164, 171–7
    axillary vein 175, 176
    closure 177
    dissection 174–5
    dressing 177
    haemostasis 177
    incision 174
    intercostobrachial nerve 175
    local draining lymph nodes 171
    long thoracic nerve of Bell 175–6
    lymphoedema risk 171
    pectoralis major 174
    postoperative seroma 177
    procedure 174–7
    review of borders 176, *177*
    stitches 177
    suction drain 177
    thoracodorsal pedicle 176

    triple assessment 171
    wound 177
axillary node sampling 172
axillary vein 175, 176

Babcock forceps 220
Bailey bone cutters 224, *225*
Bard—Parker handles 224
basilic vein graft, femorodistal bypass 89
below knee amputation 68–73
    anterior compartment muscles 70
    Burgess flap 68
    closure 72
    fibula transection 70
    gastrocnemius muscle flap 71, 72
    haemostasis 71–2
    procedure 68–72
    skew flap 68
    skin flaps 68–70
    sutures 72
    tibia division 70–1
bile duct fistula 153
bile duct T-tube 153
biliary strictures 153
Birch v UCL Hospital (2008) 248
Birkett artery forceps 219, *220*
bleeps 238–9
blood glucose 235
blood loss 234, 235
Boerhaave's syndrome 156
Bolam (and Bolitho) tests 247
bone spikes 224, *225*
bowel clamps 223, *224*
brachial artery 92–3
brachiobasilic fistula 91
brachiocephalic fistula 91–4
    anastomosis 93–4
    arteriotomy 93
    brachial artery 92–3
    duplex scan 91–2
    haemostasis 94

incision 92
median cubital vein 92
parachute technique 93–4
polytetrafluoroethylene (PTFE) graft 91
procedure 92–4
renal access 91
sutures 94
breast
axillary node clearance 164, 171–7
fibroadenoma 178–80
lactational abscess 167
latissimus dorsi flap reconstruction 176
lumpectomy 178–80
needle aspiration of abscess 167
triple assessment 171
wide local excision 166–70
cavity re-excision 169
closure 167, 169
dissection 167–8
incision 166, 167
margins 169
not palpable tumours 169
notes 169
pectoralis fascia 168
procedure 167–9
radiotherapy 169
skin flap 167–8
sutures 167, 169
wire-guided 169
see also mastectomy
breast cancer screening 169
breast implants 166
Bristow periosteal elevator 225
Burgess flap, below knee amputation 68

caecal volvulus 209
Calot's triangle 150, 151, 152
capacity
assessment 246–7
emergencies 250
patients with 247–9

patients without 249–50
potential to regain 249
carotid artery
common 74, 75, 77–8
internal 74, 75, 78
carotid endarterectomy 74–81
anaesthesia 75, 77
arteriotomy 79–80
back bleeding 80
closure 79–80
common carotid artery 77–8
evidence base 75
haemostasis 80
hypoglossal nerve 78–9
incision 77
internal carotid artery 78
landmarks 76–7
plaque 77–8
procedure 76–80
shunt 75, 79
suction drain 80
timing 75–6
transcranial Doppler 75
carpal tunnel decompression
126–9
closure 128
dressing 128
endoscopic 128
flexor retinaculum division
127, 128
incision 126–7
Kaplan's cardinal line 126, 128
median nerve 127, 128
notes 128
palmar aponeurosis 127, 128
procedure 126–8
superficial palmar arch 128
carpal tunnel syndrome 126
chest drain 158
Chester v Afshar (2004) 248
children 250–1

cholecystectomy, open 148–54
  biliary strictures 153
  Calot's triangle 150, 151, 152
  closure 152
  common hepatic duct 150, 151
  cystic artery 150, 151–2
  cystic duct 150, 151–2
  diathermy 151, 152
  endoscopic retrograde
      cholangiopancreatography 152
  gallbladder
    dissection 151
    distended 152
    hot 152–3
    location 149–50
    remnant 153
  incision 148, 149
  Kocher's incision 148
  oedematous tissue 152–3
  sutures 152
  T-tubes 153
cholecystectomy, subtotal 153
circumcision 103–6
  dressings 105
  haemostasis 105
  incision 104
  penile block 103–4
  sutures 105
colic artery 213
coliform bacteria 20
colitis, ischaemic 66
colon
  anastomosis 214
  ascending 211, 212
  carcinoma 209, 211, 212
  examination in right hemicolectomy 211
  hepatic flexure 211, 212
  sigmoid 197
  transverse 197
  tumours 209, 211, 212
colonoscopy 210

colostomy 196–200
  circular hole 198
  colon delivery 198–9
  dissection 198
  end 196
  incision 198, 199
  large bowel location 198
  loop 196, 197
    sigmoid 197–9
  marking of site 197
  procedure 197–9
  rectus sheath 198
  sigmoid colon 197–9
  sutures 199
  transverse colon 197, *199*
  trephine 197, 200
common carotid artery
  carotid endarterectomy 77–8
  stroke 74, 75
common hepatic duct 150, 151
common iliac artery 62, 63, 64
communication, theatre team 234, 238
competence, Gillick 251
Confidential Enquiry into Peri Operative Deaths
      (CEPOD) 243
consent 246–51
  emergencies 250
  paediatrics 250–1
  special circumstances 250–1
  voluntary 247
  see also capacity
consent form 232
consultant's methods 240
contraception, after vasectomy 101
Covidien™ 227
cricothyroid membrane, cannula insertion 190
cricothyroid muscle 183
cricothyroidostomy 189–90
critical events 234–5
critical limb ischaemia, femorodistal bypass 85
Crohn's disease 202

cubital vein, median 92
cutting needles 229
cystic artery 150, 151–2
cystic duct 150, 151–2
Czerny retractors 221

Deaver retractors 221
DeBakey forceps 218
deep vein thrombosis 51
dental syringe 225
dermatome 9, 10
diabetic foot abscess 20, 21
diathermy equipment 222–3
  bipolar 223
  monopolar 222–3
dietary fibre 191
discharge letter 244
dissecting scissors 219
Doppler scan
  short saphenous vein ligation 57
  transcranial for carotid endarterectomy 75
Doyen non-crushing bowel clamps
      223, *224*
drug chart 244
ductal carcinoma in situ (DCIS) 172
Dunhill artery forceps 219, *220*
duodenal ulcer
  bleeding 135, *136*
  perforated 144
duodenum
  abdominal aortic aneurysm repair 61, 62
  avoidance in right hemicolectomy 213
duplex scan
  brachiocephalic fistula 91–2
  femorodistal bypass 85, 86
  short saphenous vein ligation 57, 58
dynamic hip screw (DHS) 112–20
  closure 119
  depth gauge 119
  drilling 118–19
  insertion 118

length measurement 117
plate 118
procedure 114–19
reaming out 117–18
screwing in 118

emergencies, consent 250
endoscopic retrograde
      cholangiopancreatography (ERCP) 152
endovascular aneurysm repair (EVAR) 60
enterotomy formation 205
epididymal cysts 95–7
  closure 97
  dissection 96–7
  incision 96
epigastric artery, inferior 210
equipment, faulty 235
Ethicon™ 227
eye protection
  abscess irrigation 22
  wedge resection of ingrown toenail 24

faecal continence 191
femoral head
  avascular necrosis 112, 119
  blood supply 112
femoral hernia repair 13–19
  bowel inspection 15–16
  closure 16, 17, 18
  femoral canal repair 16, 17
  incision 13–14, 15, 17
  inguinal canal 16, 17
  Lockwood approach 13, 17–18
  Lothiessen approach 16–17
  mesh use 16, 18
  midline laparotomy 17
  modified McEvedy approach 13–16, 19
  notes 18
  peritoneum division 15, 18
  procedure 13–18
  sac 15, *16,* 17–18

femoral hernia repair (*Continued*)
  stitching 18
  sutures 16, 18
femoral neck fractures 112
  classification 113–14
  closure 119
  extracapsular 114
  fracture reduction 115
  guide pin 116–17
  hip hemiarthroplasty 121–5
  incision 115–16
  intracapsular 113–14
  muscle dissection 116
  notes 119
  plate 118
  procedure 114–19
  screw 117–18
  tip—-apex distance 117
  X-rays 115, 117
femoral pulse, abdominal aortic aneurysm
      repair 65, 66
femorodistal bypass 85–90
  anaesthesia 85
  anastomosis 88, 89
  anterior tibial artery 87
  basilic vein graft 89
  closure 89
  grafts 85, 89
  incision 86
  indications 85
  infrageniculate vessels 87
  long saphenous vein graft 85, 87–8
  notes 89
  peroneal artery 87
  polytetrafluoroethylene (PTFE) graft 85, 89
  popliteal artery 87
  posterior tibial artery 87
  preoperative scan 85, 86
  procedure 85–9
  suction drain 89
  tunnel formation 88–9

fibroadenoma 178–80
fibula, transection for below knee
      amputation 70
fistula-in-ano 20
flattened hierarchy 234
foramen of Winslow 132
forceps 218–19
  artery 219–20
  Kocher 223
  nasal 226
  tissue-holding 220–1
foreskin 104–5
foveolar artery 112

gallbladder
  dissection 151
  distended 152
  hot 152–3
  location 149–50
  remnant 153
gastrectomy 130–7
  anastomosis 134
  Billroth II 130
  duodenal stump 134–5
  foramen of Winslow 132
  gastrocolic omentum 131
  gastrojejunostomy 134
  greater omentum 133
  left gastroepiploic artery 133
  lesser omentum 133
  lesser sac 131–2
  notes 135
  omental patch repair 135
  Polya 130
  preoperative laparoscopy 131
  procedure 131–5
  pylorus 132
  right gastric artery 133
  right gastroepiploic artery 132–3
  stomach stapling 133–4
  sutures 134

gastric artery
  duodenum stapling 133
  right 133
gastric outlet lesion, obstructing 144
gastrocnemius muscle flap, below knee
    amputation 71, 72
gastrocolic omentum 131, 139, 212
gastroduodenal artery 135
gastroduodenotomy 135, *136*
gastroepiploic artery 212
  left 133
  right 132–3
gastrojejunostomy 134, 144–7
  anastomosis
    preparation 145
    procedure 145–6
  closure 146
  jejunum preparation 145
  procedure 145–6
  stapling 146
  techniques 144–5
gastrosplenic ligament 140
giant cell arteritis 82
Gillick v West Norfolk (1985) 251
Gillies forceps 218
Gillies skin hook 222
glucose, blood level 235
gonadal vein 110

haemorrhoidal artery ligation (HAL) 192
haemorrhoidectomy 191–5
  anal examination 192–3
  anal stenosis risk 194
  bleeding 193
  clips 193
  dissection 193–4
  dressing 194
  haemostasis 194
  haemostatic pack 194–5
  incision 193
  internal sphincter 194

local anaesthesia 193
Milligan—Morgan procedure 192
perianal examination 192–3
postoperative analgesia 192
procedure 192–5
retraction 193–4
stapled 192
haemorrhoids 191
  banding 192, 193
  classification 191, 192
  clips 193
  injection 192, 193
  management 191–2
haemostatic clips 219–20
hair removal 235
Hasson technique for pneumoperitoneum
    40
hemicolectomy *see* right hemicolectomy
hepatic duct, common 150, 151
hernia
  small bowel incarceration 202–3
  see also femoral hernia repair; inguinal hernia
      repair; umbilical/paraumbilical hernia
      repair
hip fractures 112
  anterolateral approach 121–5
  approaches 121
  classification 113–14
  closure 119
  displaced subcapital 119
  extracapsular 114
  fracture reduction 115
  guide pin 116–17
  incision 115–16
  intracapsular 113–14
  muscle dissection 116
  notes 119
  plate 118–19
  procedure 114–19
  screw 117–18
  tip—apex distance 117

hip fractures (*Continued*)
  total hip replacement 119
  X-rays 115, 117
  see also dynamic hip screw (DHS)
hip hemiarthroplasty 112, 113–14,
      121–5
  bony landmarks 122–3
  cemented 119, 124
  closure 125
  drapes 122
  femoral head removal 123–4
  hip relocation 124
  hip stability testing 124–5
  implant insertion 124, *125*
  implant sizing 124
  incisions 123
  muscle division 123
  procedure 121–5
  reaming of femoral shaft 124, *125*
  sterile conditions 122
  sutures 125
  Thompson 124
  thromboembolic prophylaxis 121–2
  uncemented 119, 124
hip joint, normal *113*
hip prosthesis
  Austin—Moore 124
  bipolar 119
  infections 122
Howarth elevator 224
hypersplenism 138
hypocalcaemia risk 185
hypoglossal nerve, carotid
      endarterectomy 78–9

identity confirmation of patient 232, 234
ileitis, terminal 209
ileocolic artery, right hemicolectomy 213
ileostomy 200
  end 196
  loop 196, 200

ileum
  anastomosis 214
  terminal 212
iliac artery, common 62, 63, 64
images, patient 235
Independent Mental Capacity Advocate
      (IMCA) 250
infections
  hip prosthesis 122
  see also abscess
inferior epigastric artery, ligation 210
inferior mesenteric artery 63, 66
information for patient 247–8
infrageniculate vessels, femorodistal
      bypass 87
ingrown toenail, wedge resection 24–7
inguinal hernia repair 1–7
  clips 6
  cord 2–3
  direct hernia 3, 4–5
  incision 1–2
  indirect hernia 3–4, 6
  inguinoscrotal hernia 6–7
  mesh insertion 5, 6
  notes 6–7
  procedure 1–6
  sac 2, 3, 4, 6
  staples 5–6
  stitching 5–6
  sutures 5–6
  women 6
intercostal muscles 157, 158
intercostobrachial nerve 175
intermittent claudication, femorodistal
      bypass 85
internal carotid artery
  carotid endarterectomy 78
  stroke 74, 75
intertrochanteric fracture *113*

Jenkin's rule for suture length 49

Kaplan's cardinal line 126, 128
kidney, ipsilateral agenesis 101
Killian nasal speculum 226
knot tying 239
Kocher clips 41
Kocher forceps 223

Lahey artery forceps 220
Lanes forceps 218
Lanes tissue holding forceps 220–1
Langenbeck retractors 41, 221
laparotomy 44–50
  abdominal aortic aneurysm repair 61
  abdominal content examination 47–8
  abdominal drains 48–9
  clips 46
  closure 49
  coagulating diathermy 45, 46
  incision 44, 45
  Jenkin's rule 49
  linea alba 45, 46, 49
  notes 49–50
  pelvic content examination 47–8
  preinduction antibiotics 44
  procedure 44–9
  re-do 49–50
  stoma 196, 199–200
  sutures 49
  washing out peritoneal cavity 48
laryngeal nerves
  external 183
  recurrent 183, 184–5
lasting power of attorney 250
latissimus dorsi flap, breast
     reconstruction 176
laxatives 192, 195
left renal vein 62, 66
lienorenal ligament 141
ligament of Berry 186
ligamentum teres 112
limb ischaemia, critical 85

Lockwood approach for femoral hernia repair
    13, 17–18
logbook 240
long saphenous vein graft 85, 87–8
long saphenous vein stripping 51–6
  dressings 55
  duplex scan of venous system 51
  incision 52
  ligation/division of vein tributaries 53
  marking veins 51–2
  notes 55
  procedure 51–6
  saphenofemoral junction 52
  stripppers 53–4
  sutures 55
  vein dissection 52
  vein hooks/hooking 54–5
  wound closure 55
long thoracic nerve of Bell 175–6
Lothiessen approach for femoral hernia
    repair 16–17
lumbar arteries, abdominal aortic aneurysm
    repair 63
lumpectomy 178–80
  closure 179
  dissection 179
  haemostasis 179
  incision 178–9
  sutures 179
lymph nodes
  clearance in right hemicolectomy 209, 213
  see also axillary node clearance
lymphoedema 171

malaria, splenectomised patients 139
mastectomy 160–5
  axillary node clearance 164, 171–7
  breast dissection 163
  breast identification for pathology 163–4
  closure 164
  completion 167

mastectomy (*Continued*)
    diathermy 162
    dressing 164
    incision 161
    marking breast 161
    modified radical 160
    nipple-sparing 164
    notes 164
    pectoralis fascia 163
    procedure 160–4
    prophylactic 164
    radical 160
    skin flap 161–3
    skin-sparing 164
    subcutaneous 164
    suction drain 164
    sutures 164
    synmastia 163
Mayo scissors 219
McBurney's point 37, 198
McDonald dissector 224
McEvedy approach for femoral hernia repair 13–16, 19
McIndoe double-prong skin hook 222
McIndoe forceps 218
McIndoe scissors 219
median cubital vein, brachiocephalic fistula 92
median nerve
    carpal tunnel decompression 127, 128
    recurrent motor branch 128
medication check 232
melanoma of Breslow 8–9
Mental Capacity Act (2005) 246, 249
mesenteric artery
    inferior 63, 66
    superior 202
mesher 10
metronidazole, post-haemorrhoidectomy analgesia 192
Morris retractors 221

Mosquito artery forceps 219
Moynihan artery forceps 219

nasal polyp forceps 226
nasal scissors 226
National Patient Safety Agency (NPSA) 231
needle(s) 228–9
    count 235
needle holders 221
nephrectomy 107–11
    approaches 107
    closure 110–11
    dissection 109–10
    gonadal vein 110
    incision 107, 108–9
    notes 111
    procedure 107–10, *111*
    renal artery 109–10
    renal vein 109, 110
    stitches 111
    tumour thrombus 111
    ureter 110
non-steroidal anti-inflammatory drugs (NSAIDs) 192
Norfolk and Norwich retractor 222
Northfield bone nibblers 224, *225*
nutrient artery 112

obese patients, appendicectomy 38
Omnitract retractor 61–2
oncological operations
    skin lesions 8–10
    see also mastectomy; right hemicolectomy; small bowel resection and anastomosis
operating experience 239
    discharge letter 244
operation note 240, 241, *242,* 243–5
    CEPOD list 243
    content 241, *242,* 243
    diagrams 244
    drug chart 244

elective/emergency case 243
format 243–5
handwritten 241
postoperative instructions 244
typed 241, 243
opiates, post-haemorrhoidectomy
       analgesia 192
orchidectomy 96
orchidopexy 97
orthopaedic mallet 225

paediatrics, consent 250–1
palmar arch, superficial 128
paraphimosis 103
parathyroid glands 185
paraumbilical hernia see umbilical/
       paraumbilical hernia repair
parents, consent for children 250–1
patient safety 231–2, *233*, 234–6
   identity confirmation 232, 234
patients, views of those close to 250
Pearce v United Bristol (1999) 248
pectoralis fascia 163, 168
pectoralis major 163, 172, 174
penile block 103–4
peptic ulcer, perforated 130, 135
perianal abscess 20–1
peroneal artery, femorodistal bypass 87
phenol tissue ablation 25–6
phimosis 103, 104
phrenicocolic ligament 141
piles see haemorrhoids
pilonidal sinus abscess 206, 208
pilonidal sinus excision 206–8
   bleeding 207
   closure 206, 207, 208
   diathermy 207
   granulation rosettes 207
   healing by second intention 206, 207–8
   marsupialisation 206, 208
   primary closure 206, 207, 208

skin flaps 208
sutures 207
pledgets 223
pneumoperitoneum, establishing 40–3
   camera insertion 42–3
   closure 43
   CO_2 tube 42, 43
   Hasson technique 40
   incision 41
   Kocher clips 41
   Langenbeck retractors 41
   linea alba 41, 42
   ports 42, 43
   procedure 40–3
   stitches 42
   sutures 43
   Verre's needle technique 40
polytetrafluoroethylene (PTFE) graft 91
   femorodistal bypass 85, 89
Pooles sucker 222
popliteal artery, femorodistal bypass 87
popliteal fossa 57–8
posterior tibial artery, femorodistal
       bypass 87
premorbid wishes 249
Procedure-Based Assessment (PBA) 240
procedure check 234
   name 235
proctitis 21
pyloroplasty 135, *136*

radiocephalic fistula 91
radiotherapy, breast wide local
       excision 169
Rampley sponge holder 218
Ramsey forceps 219
reasonable patient 248
recovery of patient 235
rectus sheath, posterior 210
renal access, brachiocephalic fistula 91
renal artery 109–10

renal vein 109, 110
  left 62, 66
  tumour thrombus 111
retinacular vessels 112, 114
retractors 221–2
right hemicolectomy 209–16, 214
  abdomen examination 211
  anastomosis 214, 215
  closure 215
  colic artery 213
  colon
    anastomosis 214
    ascending 211
    examination 211
    mobilisation 212–13
  colonoscopy 210
  diathermy 210
  dissection 211–12
  double-barrelled stoma 215
  duodenum avoidance 213
  emergency 215
  extended 209
  gastrocolic omentum 212
  gastroepiploic artery 212
  gonadal vessels avoidance 213
  haemostasis 215
  hand sewn 214, 215
  ileocolic artery 213
  ileum anastomosis 214
  incision 209–10
  inferior epigastric artery ligation 210
  laparoscopic 209
  lesser sac 212
  lymph node clearance 209, 213
  major vessel ligation/division 213–14
  mesenteric window 215
  notes 215
  omentum resection 214
  posterior rectus sheath 210
  procedure 209–15
  stapled 214–15

ureter avoidance 213
  white line of Toldt 211
ring-handled spikes 224, *225*
risks of surgery, warnings to patients 248–9
Roberts artery forceps 219, *220*

safety *see* patient safety
saphenopopliteal junction 57, 58
scissors 219
  nasal 226
scrotal examination 95–8
  epididymal cysts 95–7
scrubs 238, 239
sentinel lymph node biopsy 172
shin, skin lesions 8
short saphenous vein ligation 57–9
  closure 58–9
  incision 57
  preoperative scan 57, 58
  sutures 59
shunt, carotid endarterectomy 75, 79
Sidaway v Bethlem Royal Hospital (1985) 248
skew flap, below knee amputation 68
skin flaps
  below knee amputation 68–70
  breast wide local excision 167–8
  mastectomy 161–3
  pilonidal sinus excision 208
skin hooks 222
small bowel
  adhesions 202, 205
  incarceration in hernia 202–3
  inflammation 202
  lymphoma 202
  tumours 202
  viability assessment 202–3
  volvulus 202
small bowel resection and anastomosis 202–5
  anastomosis formation 204–5
  anastomotic leak 203
  dehiscence 203

enterotomy formation 205
hand sewn 203
incision 203
ischaemia 203, 206
  risk 205
mesenteric window
  closure 206
  formation 204
mesentery inspection 203
procedure 203–5
stapled 203
stapling 205
sutures 205–6
wound protection 205
specimens, labelling 235
Spencer-Wells artery forceps
        219, 220
spleen
  abscess 138
  bleeding control 143
  conservative surgery 143
  cysts 138
  iatrogenic damage 139
  trauma 139, 142–3
splenectomy 138–43
  delivery of spleen 141–2
  gastrocolic omentum 139
  gastrosplenic ligament 140
  incisions 139
  indications
    elective 138
    emergency 139
  information about state 139
  lienorenal ligament 141
  notes 142–3
  phrenicocolic ligament 141
  procedure 139–42
  prophylactic antibiotics 139
  splenic artery 139–40, 141, 142
    division 141–2
  splenic vein 142

splenocolic ligament 140
trauma 139, 142–3
vaccinations 139
splenic artery 139–40, 141, 142
  division 141–2
splenic vein 142
  thrombosis 138
splenocolic ligament 140
splenunculi 142
split skin graft 8–12
  anaesthesia 9, 11
  contraindications 11
  dressings 11
  glue 11
  graft application 10–11
  graft preparation 10
  harvesting 9–10
  indications 8–9
  notes 11
  procedure 9–11
  staples 11
  sutures 11
sterile field 238
sternotomy, median 155
steroids, giant cell arteritis 82
Stevens crushing bowel clamps
        223, 224
stitch-cutting scissors 219
stoma 196–200
  double-barrelled 215
stoma bag 199
stoma care nurse 197
stroke
  common carotid artery 74, 75
  internal carotid artery 74, 75
  ischaemic 74
suckers 222
superior mesenteric artery, emboli 202
superior thyroid artery 182, 183
supralevator induration 21
surgical errors 231–2

surgical instruments 217–26
  Bard—Parker handles 224
  bowel clamps 223, *224*
  count 235
  diathermy equipment 222–3
  ENT 225–6
  forceps 218–19
    artery 219–20
    Kocher 223
    nasal 226
    tissue-holding 220–1
  haemostatic clips 219–20
  Howarth elevator 224
  McDonald dissector 224
  nasal speculum 226
  needle holders 221
  orthopaedic 224–5
  retractors 221–2
  scissors 219
    nasal 226
  skin hooks 222
  sponge holder 218
  suckers 222
  Volkmann spoon 224
Surgical Site Infection Bundle 235
sustentaculum lienis 141
sutures 227–30, 229
  absorbable 228, 229, *230*
  braided 228
  Caprosyn 229, *230*
  Ethilon *230*
  Maxon 229, *230*
  Monocryl 229, *230*
  monofilament 228
  Monosof *230*
  needle type 228–9
  non-absorbable 228, 229–30
  nylon 230
  PDS 229, *230*
  Permahand silk *230*
  polyfilament 228

  Polysorb 229, *230*
  Prolene 229–30
  silk 230
  size 228
  Sofsilk *230*
  Surgipro 229–30
  thickness 228
  Vicryl 229, *230*
swab-on-a-stick 218
swabs, count 235
synmastia 163

T-tube, bile duct 153
tapercut needles 229
temperature, patient 235
temporal artery biopsy 82–4
  closure 84
  dressings 84
  incision 83
  marking of temporal artery 82–3
  procedure 82–4
  sutures 84
tension pneumothorax 158
terminal ileitis 209
terminal ileum 212
testis
  examination 96, 99
  torsion 97
theatre etiquette 237–40
  after operation 240
  assisting 239
  awake patient 239–40
  basic skills 239
  bleeps 238–9
  cleaning up 240
  consultant's methods 240
  debrief with trainer 240
  dress 238
  groundwork 237
  operating experience 239
  during operation 239–40

usefulness 238, 239, 240
theatre team 234, 238
  thanks to 240
thoracodorsal pedicle 176
thoracotomy 155–9
  analgesia 159
  anterolateral 155
  approaches 155–6
  chest drain 158
  clamshell 155
  closure 158–9
  incision 156–7
  intercostal muscles 157, 158
  intercostal space approach 157
  left lateral 155
  pleural lining 157
  posterolateral 155
  procedure 156–9
  ribs 157, 158, 159
  sutures 158–9
  thoracoabdominal 156
  wound pain 159
thromboembolic deterrent stockings
    (TEDS) 235
thyroid artery
  inferior 185
  superior 182, 183
thyroid veins 182
thyroidectomy 181–6
  cricothyroid muscle 183
  diathermy 185–6
  dissection 182
  dressing 186
  haemostasis 186
  hoarse voice risk 183, 184
  hypocalcaemia risk 185
  incision 181–2
  laryngeal nerves 183, 184–5
  ligament of Berry 186
  parathyroid glands 185
  procedure 181–6

suction drain 186
  thyroid arteries 182, 183, 185
  thyroid veins 182
tibia, division for below knee amputation 70–1
tibial artery, anterior/posterior 87
Tilley—Henkel forceps 226
tissue-holding forceps 220–1
toenail, ingrown, wedge resection 24–7
toee hammer 225–6
total hip replacement 119
tracheostomy 187–90
  haemostasis 188
  incision 187–8
  location 188, *189*
  non-permanent 189
  notes 189–90
  percutaneous 187
  procedure 187–9
  stitching 189
  strap muscles 188
  taping to neck 189
  trachea opening 189
tracheostomy tube 188–9
transcranial Doppler, carotid
    endarterectomy 75
transfer of patient 240, 244
transient ischaemic attacks (TIAs) 74
Travers retractor 222
tumour thrombus, renal vein 111

umbilical/paraumbilical hernia repair 28–33
  anatomy 28
  clips 31
  incidence of hernias 28
  incision 29, 32
  Mayo repair 30–1
  mesh use 30, 31–2
  notes 32
  peritoneal sac 29, 30
  procedure 29–32
  skin resection 32

umbilical/paraumbilical hernia repair
(*Continued*)
  sutures 30–1, 32
  umbilical cicatrix 30
  umbilicus reconstruction 32
  vest-over-pants repair 30–1
ureter 110

varicose veins, long saphenous vein
stripping 51–6
vas deferens 100–1
  unilateral agenesis 101
vasectomy 99–102
  contraception 101
  haemostasis 101
  incision 100
  ligation of vas 100–1
  notes 101–2
  procedure 99–101
  reversal 101–2
  scalpel-free technique 101
  sperm count 101
venous thromboembolism 235
Verre's needle technique for
pneumoperitoneum 40

visiting patient 240
Volkmann spoon 224

warnings to patients of risks 248–9
wedge resection of ingrown toenail 24–7
  closure 26
  dressings 26
  incision 25
  notes 26
  phenol ablation 25–6
  procedure 24–6
  simple avulsion 26
  Zadek's procedure 26
West retractor 222
white line of Toldt 211
WHO Surgical Safety Checklist 232, *233*,
234–5, 239
  sign in 232, *233*, 234
  sign out *233*, 235
  time out *233*, 234–5
women, inguinal hernia repair 6

Yankauer sucker 222

Zadek's procedure 26